# A Taoist Guide to Longevity

# A Taoist Guide to Longevity

*Bian Zhizhong*

*Translated by Liu Zongren*

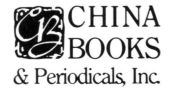

CHINA
BOOKS
& Periodicals, Inc.

Cover and interior design by Linda Revel

Illustrations by Wu Tianda

Edited by Fan Zhilong and Bob Schildgen

Library of Congress Catalog Card Number: 89-60881
ISBN 0-8351-2277-8

Printed in the United States of America

Published in the United States of America by CHINA
BOOKS
& Periodicals, Inc.

# Contents

Acknowledgements        7
Preface        9
Introduction        11

Exercise 1:  Restoring Spring        20
Exercise 2:  Vital Energy        22
Exercise 3:  The Eight Diagrams        26
Exercise 4:  Roc Flying        30
Exercise 5:  Turtle Retracting Its Head        32
Exercise 6:  The Swimming, Smiling Dragon        36
Exercise 7:  Frog Swimming        40
Exercise 8:  Heaven Circles and Earth Circles        42
Exercise 9:  Ren Rings        44
Exercise 10:  Phoenix Spreads Its Wings        50
Exercise 11:  Rejuvenating the Face        52
Exercise 12:  Transverse Circles        60
Exercise 13:  Vertical Circles        61
Exercise 14:  Horizontal Circles        62

More About the Exercises        63
Point Diagrams        66

# Acknowledgements

I was encouraged to make these exercises public principally by Dr. M. C. Niu, a Chinese-American biologist; Xu Renhe, former president of Beijing's Guanganmen Hospital; Zhang Dianhua, former director of the Acupuncture Research Institute; and Tao Jiashan from the Beijing Physical Culture and Sports Commission. During the process of sorting out the material and compiling it into a book I received great help from my Taoist friends, colleagues, students, and especially Mr. Sun Tao and Mr. Wu Zonghai of Hong Kong.

This book is the result of collective wisdom. I would like to take this opportunity to express my sincere thanks to these people. They have the same wishes as mine: good health and long life to all the world's people.

—*Bian Zhizhong,*
**President, Ancient Chinese Health
Preservation Research Institute,
Beijing**

# Preface

Bian Zhizhong is a quiet man living a quiet life. Now in his seventies, he is strong, agile and flexible, his skin glows, and he is in excellent health. This alone is testimony to the benefits of the exercises in this book. As a young man, Mr. Bian met a Taoist abbot of the Huashan Mountains school who taught him these exercises. This was before Liberation (1949), and the Taoists were very strict about their prohibition: "No passing on to either parents or children." So Mr. Bian practiced these exercises on his own for forty years. But as the years passed, many Taoist secret practices were being made public. Some people learned of the advanced practices without mastering the basic practices that preceded them.

Mr. Bian felt that people needed to build their practice on a solid foundation. Therefore, he decided to offer these exercises to the public through articles as well as personal instruction.

"All the Huashan Mountains School Taoists who had mastered these exercises had died, and I was approaching seventy. If I couldn't make these exercises known to the public, they might be lost forever and the painstaking efforts of many centuries of Taoists would be in vain," he has said.

The enthusiastic response to his exercises confirmed the correctness of this decision. People from the far reaches of China read his articles, learned the exercises, and wrote letters of praise for their power.

Mr. Bian is the successor to a long line of Taoist wisdom that is now being seriously studied in China.

# Introduction

The exercises described in this book are the foundation of a larger system first developed by Taoist monks well over a thousand years ago. These particular exercises are from the All True Branch of the Huashan Mountain School, which was established in the Qin dynasty (1115–1234) and were passed down over the centuries orally and in secret. For a brief period in China's long history, the monks of Huashan Mountain enjoyed the patronage of the emperors, but due to changing political circumstances they were forced to practice in obscurity for many centuries.

Taoist health practices have their roots in prehistoric healing methods which date as far back as 4,000 years, when tribal peoples in China used breathing and dance exercises to relieve illnesses. By the sixth century B.C., scholars had begun to classify and discuss various methods of movement and breathing for health maintenance. Illustrations of the movements, carved in jade, survive from this period.

Continuing attention over the centuries developed the theory and practice, often in close association with Traditional Chinese Medicine, which discovered the importance of the flow through the body of the vital energy force known as *qi*. Famous Taoists were also practicioners of medicine, developing acupuncture, herbalism, and exercises into a complex system. A book discovered in an archaeological dig, entitled *Dao Ying Qi Fa* (The Way to Induce Free Qi Flow), and dating back to the Western Han dynasty (206 B.C.–A.D. 24) actually contains illustrations of exercises remarkably similar to those practiced to this day. Hua Tuo, the renowned doctor-herbalist-acupuncturist in the Eastern Han dynasty (A.D. 25–220), was also famed for his health preservation exercises. His sayings "The door hinge is never worm-eaten" and "running water never gets stale" sum up the relation between Taoist exercises and longevity.

In the Eastern Han dynasty, Taoism became an established religion. With its emphasis on the here-and-now, a basic tenet of Taoism is to seek well-being and happiness while attempting to attain immortality. The cultivation of physical health and longevity therefore were central to its philosophical system. It also absorbed ideas from Buddhism and Confucianism. For another six centuries, Taoism was in favor with the emperors, who began to use it for their own political purposes. Like other religions, it also absorbed superstitions and rituals which tended to obscure its basic ideas. The emperors of the Tang Dynasty (A.D. 618–907) were open to the use of Taoist exercises for health maintenance and prevention of disease.

With the changing dynasties, imperial support for Taoism ended, and practices had to be carried on in secret, with esoteric teachings passed down orally from generation to generation. It was only after Liberation (1949) that the code of silence was broken and this ancient wisdom about chaneling the body's energy, breathing, and meditation began to be brought to the public.

## Holistic Approach

Although Taoism became entangled in political matters and superstitious practices, its core teaching on health maintenance remains scientifically sound.

At the root of these Taoist methods is a holistic approach, which maintains that all the body's organs are interrelated and that a condition in one organ may be caused by the malfunction of another organ or a blockage in the flow of the body's energy. The Taoists also realized that the mind and body were profoundly interrelated, and that attitudes and emotional states could influence one's physical condition and that the body's organs could affect psychological conditions. While some of their terminology may seem rather quaint by modern standards, the Taoists' basic approach has been corroborated by modern science. For example, our knowledge of the endocrine system shows just how closely interrelated different parts of the body are. And the fields of nutrition, internal medicine and psychiatry provide ample evidence of the complex interdependence of body and mind. Indeed, modern discoveries in biochemistry and neurophysiology have demonstrated that the "physical" and "psychological" are more intimately bound together than ever suspected. The mind-body dualism, for centuries a basic assumption in the West, has been discredited by the West's own science, to be replaced by a view more akin to the holistic concepts of the Taoists.

As noted, the Taoist approach to health closely follows the development of Traditional Chinese Medicine. In fact, it is often difficult to separate the contributions of the Taoists and the physicians—in many cases the physicians were Taoists and vice versa.

Traditional Chinese medicine stands today as a unique holistic system that includes acupuncture, herbs, and exercises. The exercises in this book will take on a deeper meaning when the roots of the system are better understood.

## The Taoist World View and the Concept of Yin-Yang

All people have developed explanations of how the universe began, how the world was formed and how life and humanity emerged. The ancient Taoists, careful observers of nature, concluded that the primal substance of the universe is qi (prounounced "chi"). It can be translated as "vital energy" or "vital force" or "breath," especially in the sense of "breath of life." (The West, too, expresses this concept of vital energy in similar terms: the word "spirit," used to describe a vital force running through body, mind, and universe, is derived from the Latin for "wind" or "breath." The

image of wind on the waters in Genesis or the idea of God "breathing" "life" into Adam are mythical attempts to express this). In the beginning, the Taoists say, there was only qi. Then the primordial qi divided into heaven and earth, the first duality or pair of opposites.

This pair of opposites was called *yin* and *yang*. In this case, yin stands for earth and yang for heaven. Yin also stands for the moon, water, cold, dark, and the shady side of the hill, while yang stands for the sun, fire, heat, light and the sunny side of the hill. The Taoists then found that everything in nature could be seen in terms of yin and yang. The concept of yin and yang is a concept of change. Day and night take their turn; the energies in the body wax and wane. So the idea of balance is that yin and yang are in their proper proportions and ebb and flow at the right times.

The symbol of yin-yang (see cover illustration) embodies the fluid nature of yin and yang. The dark and light sectors representing yin and yang are enclosed in the same circle. Not only do they change into each other but the yin contains a little bit of yang, and the yang contains some yin. This means that nothing is purely yin or yang but has traces of its opposite in its very nature. The light dot in the yin side and the dark dot in the yang side further emphasize this reality.

## "Daily" Qi, Jing (Prenatal) Qi, and Sexual Energy

Because all of nature is made up of qi, we derive our qi from the food we eat and the air we breathe. Then, like the animals, we have to rest to assimilate and distribute the qi in the body. This qi, which could be called the "daily" qi, is responsible for most of our daily activities: eating, digesting, breathing, thinking, walking, talking, and even reading this book. It is also called "postnatal qi," because it is absorbed after we are born.

The Taoists also identified another kind of qi in the body, called *jing qi,* or *yuan qi,* most commonly translated as "prenatal qi" or "congenital qi." The jing qi is present at birth as a kind of inborn vitality, a life force, a sense of energy given to every human being. This jing qi, however, is considered to be finite, and when it is completely consumed, death results. Proper use of exercise and breathing, however, can preserve this vital force. Various techniques can guide its flow through the body and harmonize it with postnatal qi, making it possible to maintain optimum health, slow down the aging process, and lengthen life. The point of the exercises is to prevent the qi from being blocked and to let it flow unobstructed through the body. If it is blocked, it cannot effectively maintain vitality. This makes the body vulnerable to all diseases, speeding up the aging process.

The jing qi is stored in the Kidney. By "Kidney," the Chinese mean the *Xiadan,* the entire lower abdominal and pubic area where jing qi resides. The Huashan Mountain School places more emphasis on activating the qi in this area than some other schools. The Kidney, in Chinese medicine, also has a special relationship with the bones, teeth, brain, hair of the head, and endocrine system, as well as the sexual and reproductive functioning. The ears are the sense organ related to the Kidney. Therefore, exercises to help arthritis, poor memory, ringing in the ears, or impotence would all be exercises that benefit the Kidney and help preserve the jing qi. Sexual functioning is entirely dependent on jing qi, and the jing qi itself is regarded as the source of sperm, ova, and sexual arousal.

Although the prenatal qi is limited, many who practice the discipline of *qigong* (which means "qi cultivation") believe it helps restore some amount of lost jing qi. They maintain that this regenerative power explains why qigong helps people recover from disease and gives them a feeling of rejuvenation.

## The Role of Sexual Exercises in Chinese Medicine

Since the amount of prenatal qi was seen as limited, its conservation became an important goal. Chinese medicine maintained that men lost their major allotment of jing qi through ejaculation and women lost their jing qi through menstruation and childbirth. But it is possible to learn techniqes to retain this energy in the body and tap its healing power.

One way to get this healing energy is by tranforming sexual qi into "daily" qi. This gives the body another source of energy.

The Taoists developed exercises to strengthen the glands and organs. By developing the qi in each organ, they would be less dependent on jing qi for their functioning and reach a higher level of health and well-being.

Many of the exercises in this book use twisting and bending exercises at the waist to strengthen the Kidney system directly by giving it an internal massage.

Some exercises stimulate the gonads directly by squeezing the thighs together. In women, squeezing the vulva stimulates the vaginal walls to secrete lubricative fluid. For men, squeezing the thighs together directly stimulates the testicles.

For both men and women, the muscles along the pelvic floor and those of the urogenital diaphragm are exercised. Strengthening the pelvic floor helps give better support to all the internal organs. Vitalizing all the organs while conserving and activating qi helps prevent sagging of the skin and internal organs, a common sign of aging.

## Avoiding Chronic Diseases

Although the average lifespan in many nations has been steadily increasing, for millions of people this longer life only means a longer period of declining health and suffering. The chronic diseases of old age plague us as much as ever.

In traditional Chinese medicine, growth, development and aging of the body is considered closely related to Kidney vitality. With strong Kidney vitality, you will age slowly, stay healthy in your old age, and live to a ripe old age. Indeed, modern science's resarch on the "biological clock" of cells indicates that there may be no biological reason why most people could not live to the age of 100 or more.

Western medicine has found that sex hormones and other hormones play an important role in maintaining normal functions of all the organs in the body. Further, current research is showing that stress is really a major cause of disease, gradually wearing down the body's resistance. But the Western tradition does not offer people a complete system which mobilizes the body's own inner resources to restore and maintain health and vitality. Qigong can be used fill this gap in Western medicine.

By its very nature, qigong is healing: it produces a calm, peaceful, optimistic outlook, a grace in movement, and a joyful disposition. The Huashan Mountain exercises, with their emphasis on Kidney function, increase Kidney vitality, thereby deterring aging and promoting health. To further understand how this works, we need to take a brief look at the relation between Taoist exercises and the theory of acupuncture in traditional Chinese medicine.

## An Energy Map of the Body: Channels (Meridians), Acupuncture and Points

The first book on the subject of medicine, called the Neijing, *The Yellow Emperor's Classic of Internal Medicine,* was compiled somewhere between 1000 B.C. and 200 B.C. These dates represent the range of scholars' opinions. However, by the time it was written down it had already evolved into a complete system of diagnosis and treatment.

The methods of diagnosis discussed in the Neijing are still used today by traditional practitioners. They include the correlation of many factors such as a person's health history, recent exposure to wind, cold, heat, wet, or dry, as well as current mental attitude and any extremes of emotion. These supplement diagnosis by the physical evidence from examination of the pulses at the wrist and the other clues on the tongue and face. Over the centuries, medical knowledge was researched and expanded.

According to Chinese Medicine theory, the energy in the body, the qi, flows in specific patterns. Twelve meridians or channels, identified as the pathways, form an energy map of the body. Ten of the meridians are associated with five pairs of organs; the other two meridians describe functions rather than organs.

The five major organs and their associated organs are:

> Lung/Large Intestine
> Liver/Gall Bladder
> Kidney/Urinary Bladder
> Heart/Small Intestine
> Spleen (Stomach)/Pancreas

The two other meridians, the Pericardium and the Triple Burner, harmonize the functioning of all the organs.

The twelve meridians originate or end at the fingertips and toes and travel to and from the organs along defined pathways. Each meridian goes to its internal organ but travels beneath the skin. By inserting a slender needle into a specific point on the skin, a meridian can be activated that will send more energy to the particular organ to restore its functioning. For a "map" of the points and channels affected by exercises in this book, see pages 66–69.

The action of the needle is somewhat like a "Roto-rooter"—it breaks up blockages (congestion) so that energy then shoots through the meridian and clears the channel.

## Acupuncture and Modern Science

Although the workings of this energy system are not yet understood by modern science, the tangible *results* of acupuncture have been accepted in many areas. For example, the Harvard Medical College operates The Pain and Stress Relief Clinic at Lemuel Shattuck Hospital, where acupuncture is one of the main treatments.

Perhaps the most convincing testimony to the effectiveness of acupuncture is its successful use in animals. The ability of acupuncture to heal animals obviously cannot be attributed to "psychological" causes or the placebo effect. In fact, veterinary research may turn out to be the key to raising the acceptance of acupuncture among doctors and scientists in the United States.

The use of acupuncture for treating infertility in cows, back pain in horses and post-surgical recovery in horses, and many common problems of cats and dogs is documented in veterinary journals. Although these techniques were developed in China, they are being tested and incorporated with increasing frequency to maintain the health of livestock in Europe and the United States. In 1975, the International Veterinary Acupuncture society was established and now has over 200 members. The society conducts a certification program for members.

Even the American Veterinary Medical Association has indicated that veterinary acupuncture and acutherapy are valid methods of treatment. The official position of the AMVA is that acupuncture procedures should be regulated by state veterinary laws just as the more conventional treatments for animals.

## Exercise to Benefit the Organs

Acupuncture and acupressure are methods used to *treat* diseases by stimulating energy flow and relieving blockages and imbalances. Taoist exercises, however, are designed to *prevent* blockages and encourage energy flow *before* symptoms of disease appear. Instead of waiting until illness breaks out and then applying acupuncture for relief, the practice of Taoist exercises stimulates points to ward off the disorder in the first place. Therefore, the exercises are a type of preventive medicine, a way of *maintaining* health by using the same basic principles as acupuncture and acupressure. The difference is that they attempt to maintain the body in a condition where acupuncture does not need to be used as a cure. But like acupuncture, the exercises can also be used to help remedy diseases and hasten recovery.

Although much has been accomplished using the external energy of acupuncture and herbs to harmonize the energy in the body, qigong experts declare that the best person to control your energy is yourself, through disciplined movements and breathing. Your own vital energy, your qi, is available to you twenty-four hours a day. When you know how to use it properly you can restore your own health, prevent future illness, and open up the possibilities of a longer, more vigorous life.

Moving the body in a specific way to stimulate a point may seem rather indirect and not very powerful, but it is exactly this subtlety that is its power. It is the power of wind and water to clean and scour and reshape the landscape.

## Taoist Exercises and the Heart

The Kidney and the Heart have a special relationship. The Kidney element is water, the Heart element is fire. It is important that the fire and the water be in proper proportion to avoid the water putting out the fire or the fire vaporizing all the water. That is why many of the exercises described here will also balance the Kidney and Heart energy.

Many types of exercises aim at improved circulation and well-being by moving an increased amount of oxygen to the cells of the body and expanding the blood vessels through vigorous activity and intensified heart action.

Rather than achieving these effects through strenuous movement, these traditional Taoist exercises rely on relaxation to achieve the dilation of the peripheral capillaries to carry more oxygenated blood to the cells. In this sense, the exercises could be called "aerobic." It is typical that while practicing these slow-moving exercises the breathing slows down and the hands get warm, red and slightly swollen as more blood is being carried to the cells. Some teachers say that you should feel so relaxed while moving that a mosquito would not be able to get a foothold and would just slide off your skin.

Because of this relaxing effect, the exercises described here have helped many people with high blood pressure as well as heart disease. The combination of relaxation and increased circulation of blood could help prevent stroke and hardening of the arteries. Of course the exercises are able to relieve any type of tension in the body and produce a feeling of calm and concentration.

## Qigong in China Today

Qigong is a general term for traditional Chinese cultivation of powers residing in the body: it includes everything from breaking cement blocks with your head to sitting in meditation. The major emphasis of the qigong in this book is on health and longevity: both treatment and prevention of disorders that lead to aging or are symptoms of aging.

In China, people can learn qigong at school, at workers' clubs, and even from teachers in the park. In the hospitals of Traditional Chinese Medicine qigong is sometimes part of the prescription for the patient.

For many sick people in China, qigong is still used only as a last resort. Having tried both Western and Chinese traditional medicines, they find themselves close to giving up and are willing to try qigong. They generally have chronic problems, such as arthritis, bone and joint diseases, high blood pressure, digestive disorders, and lung problems. There are even special qigong exercises for treating cancer.

For others, various forms of qigong have become a routine method of helping to maintain health. Early in the morning, many people in the parks and on sidewalks can be seen practicing some variety of qigong exercise, with the younger people doing the more demanding exercises while the elderly appreciate the slower movements. One of the reasons for the rapid spread of these exercises is their effectiveness. People know from personal experience how effective the breathing, movement and massage described here can be.

## How to Use This Book
The exercises in this book do not require any paraphernalia nor do they take up much space when they are being carried out. An area as big as yourself with your arms spread out is sufficient, and the exercises may be done indoors or out, at any time. Some of the sitting exercises may even be carried out while working, reading, or doing various tasks while seated.

The majority of the exercises in this book are done standing. However, for those who cannot stand, or cannot stand for long periods, most of the standing exercises can be adapted to a sitting posture—especially Frog Swimming, Heaven Circles, Earth Circles, Ren Rings, and Moistening the Skin.

Each of the exercises in this book is followed by a section called "Benefits." The benefits are described in both modern and traditional Chinese medical terms. You will find a list, in modern medical terms, of disorders which can be alleviated by the exercises. Along with this is a list of points that are stimulated by the exercise.

The points are identified by their Chinese name in pinyin romanization which describes something about them. For instance, *Xuehai* means the "Sea of Blood"; *Mingmen* means "vital gate." They will also be identified using a Western system, which includes the name of the meridian and the number assigned to the point, such as "Large Intestine—4."

It is difficult to learn movement exercises simply from the written word and two-dimensional illustrations. However, even if you only approximate a movement at first, you will still benefit from doing it.

We have attempted to make it as easy as possible to use by having a large page format and  printing each set of instructions and illustrations on facing pages. These features allow you to refer to the drawings without the inconvenience and delay of paging around in the book to find the illustration to which the text refers.  This will also make it easier to concentrate more fully on the movements themselves.

*Patience* is extremely important in becoming adept at these exercises. As in learning any unfamiliar movement, be it a dance step or a sport maneuver, slow deliberate practice is required. Remember, rushing the exercises is the very opposite of spirit of calm which they are intended to produce. Sometimes the learning process will require going back over steps that are unclear at first, looking at the drawings again and rereading the instructions. With a reasonable amount of effort and careful repetition you will learn the movements so well that they will become almost automatic.

## Becoming Aware of Your Internal Energy
At first, you will be concerned with mastering the exercises and learning them well enough so that you don't need to refer to the book at each step. Once you have learned an exercise, you will find that you can relax more as you do

it. Concentration and relaxation go hand in hand. The more you can relax and concentrate on the exercise the more acute your awareness of your own energy will become. The more effortless the movements themselves become, the more you can focus attention into your body and its energy flows.

As you do the exercise you may notice your hands getting warm or a lightness or tingling in your body during certain exercises. Other signs might be: numbness, heat, vibrating or humming feeling. Sometimes the energy enters an area that has been previously congested or covered with scar tissue. When this happens there may be momentary pain, feeling like an electric shock or intense heat, or a sensation of ants biting you. Any one of these indicates that energy is moving. Practice attentiveness and watch inside the body to feel the warm flow of energy through the channels.

## Stop When You Feel Good

The Taoist system maintains that the organs, not the brain, are responsible for your emotions. When the organs are healthy a person feels good, makes sound decisions and achieves a sense of emotional and physical well-being and a clarity of thought. The negative emotions are considered the internal cause of disease. When a person is angry, sad, worried, impatient or frightened, the emotion is being generated in an organ and is also damaging that organ and the organs related to it.

Aside from improving health and longer life, one simple yet important purpose of the exercises in this book is to *give you a glowing sense of well-being*. Therefore, if after a specific exercise you feel light-hearted, calm, relaxed and mellow, then you've accomplished enough: you don't necessarily have to proceed to another set. The exercise has achieved its benefit.

Your organs are now in harmony and you feel you can go about your daily tasks with a new attitude of involvement and pleasure. In this manner you can decide how many exercises you wish to do in a day. You can rotate through the exercises, doing one or two each day, however you like.

## Smile

This is a unique request. The practices of many qigong schools only demand a serious focusing of attention, usually at the lower abdomen. But if you can develop a child's mind of openness, curiosity and delight in simple pleasures, the nervous system is stimulated in a beneficial way: breathing becomes more even, limbs move freely, and the exercises feel light. You are able to experience your own energy more clearly.

## Round and Soft Movement Is the Key

In every exercise, the arms, shoulders or trunk are describing an arc or a circle. When moving in any direction, try to feel that the muscles are relaxed and that the exercise is effortless. Roundness in the exercises helps promote the flow of qi. You will become more adept at smoothing the motions as you progress in practice. The speed of the exercises is also a matter of practicing until you find a speed that is best for you personally. It is important, however, never to rush through the movements.

## Don't Practice Right After Eating

The exercises can be practiced at any time. It is traditional to practice them in the morning after getting up or in the evening before going to sleep, but almost anytime except immediately before or after meals is fine. You should wait at least an hour after eating to begin a session. Note that pregnant women are cautioned not to engage in several of the movements.

There is so much individual variation that it is impossible to prescribe a time of day for the exercises. The key is to find which times work best for *you* both in terms of your schedule and the amount of benefit gained at a given time. Part of the process of learning the exercises is learning more about yourself. As you progress, you will discover what times and what exercises are most beneficial for you.

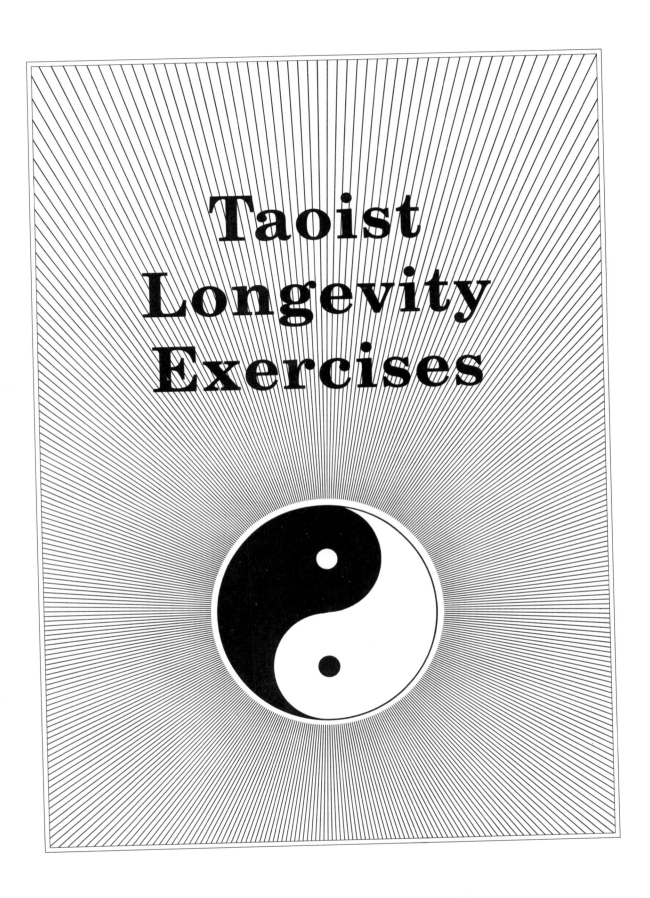

# Taoist Longevity Exercises

# Exercise 1: Restoring Spring (Nourishing the Kidney through Breathing)

## Breathing While Rising on the Toes

*By "kidney," the Chinese aren't referring to the organ itself, but to the lower abdominal region and the energy residing there.*

### Opening Posture

Stand with the legs shoulder-width apart, back straight and muscles relaxed, arms relaxed at the sides, palms toward the thighs. Relax all muscles, look straight ahead relaxing the eyes, and try to empty your mind of thoughts and images (**fig. 1**).

the abdomen to help expel the breath. Then let the chest sink and relax and shoulders slightly round while descending. As the heels make contact with the ground, let the relaxation continue as the knees bend slightly (**fig. 3**).

### Points of Attention

By pulling in the abdomen during exhalation, the lungs are emptied more efficiently, creating more room in them for the next inhalation. On inhaling, feel the fresh air and fresh energy filling the entire body. Let yourself feel the air flowing all the way down to the toes on the inhale and watch for a gentle, relaxed feeling on the exhale as the body begins to assimilate the new energy.

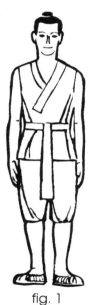 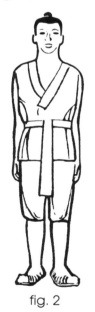

fig. 1      fig. 2

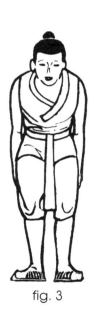 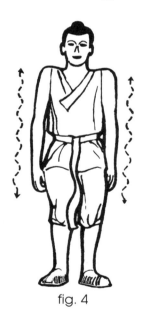

fig. 3      fig. 4

### Movements

Inhale while rising up slowly on the toes and balls of the feet, raising the heels only as far as you feel balanced. In breathing, allow the abdomen to swell outward to bring more air deep into the lungs (**fig. 2**), and continue filling the lungs by expanding the chest. This breathing should be in one easy, continuous motion.

Exhale slowly while bringing the heels back to the ground. While exhaling, contract

Repeat this sequence sixteen times.

### Shaking the Body

After the last exhalation, relax the body completely, arms relaxed at the sides, knees bent slightly, and shake the body all over at the same time in a springing vibration (**fig. 4**). Men should feel the testicles swinging slightly. Women should feel the vagina relaxed and slightly open and the breasts jiggling. All the muscles of the body should be involved in this shaking and vibrating so that even the teeth click as the jaw relaxes. With increasing experience even the internal organs are felt shaking.

Continue shaking vigorously for about a minute. The breathing during the shaking will take care of itself. Concentrate on the different parts of the body during the shaking.

If you feel stiff and have trouble starting the shaking, you can move the upper body back and forth or side to side or even shimmy to start the shaking. Some people find that if they stand still for a few minutes and try to relax as completely as possible, feeling the feet supporting all the weight of the body, shaking will start spontaneously.

## Loosening the Back and Squeezing the Organs

After shaking, check your stance and make sure your feet are still shoulder-width apart, and shift your weight to the front part of your feet, relaxing the entire body. Bend your knees, relax the jaw and tongue, and let the arms hang loosely, like ropes, moved by the actions of the trunk and shoulders. Breathing will become regulated and rhythmic on its own, with no special pattern required.

Bring the right shoulder forward, right knee dipping just slightly, twisting to the left

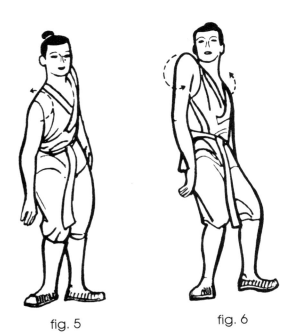

fig. 5          fig. 6

at the waist. Continue slowly, bringing the shoulder forward and up in a circle and then lowering it backward, letting the shoulder blades come together, as your left shoulder is brought forward naturally by this movement **(fig. 5)**. Keep lifting the left shoulder, making the same type of circle going forward, up, over and back while twisting the waist to the right. As the left shoulder is going up and back, let the right shoulder come forward again **(fig. 6)**. In this way you are alternately bringing the left and right shoulders forward. The twisting of the waist is beneficial, and as much attention should be paid to this part of the exercise as in tracing the circles with the shoulders.

Repeat sixteen times.

Do not strain or overexert, because the shoulder movements need not be large at first. Continued practice of the shoulder movements will gradually increase mobility and result in the ability to make larger circles.

## Benefits

Restoring Spring is the foundation for the rest of the exercises. It absorbs fresh energy, expels stale air and toxins in the body, regulates the internal organs, stimulates the circulation of qi and blood, and increases vitality.

The continuous twisting of the torso squeezes the internal organs, giving them a gentle massage and improving their function. Any movement of gas—belching, farting, bubbling or rumbling sounds—is a good sign and should be welcomed.

This movement eases shoulder and back pain, abdominal distension and menstrual pain. It also helps in weight reduction, sexual dysfunction and weakness in general.

It is recommended that beginners learn Restoring Spring thoroughly and practice it twice a day, three to five minutes each time. When you become proficient at it and have begun to feel some benefits, then proceed to Movement 2: Vital Energy (Squeezing the Yin).

# Exercise 2: Vital Energy (Squeezing the Yin)

*This exercise is the same for men and women, and strengthens the muscles of the pelvic floor, which support all the internal organs. The movements especially vitalize the sexual organs and glands. Although the movements are the same for men and women, in Chinese the men's exercise is called "Squeezing the Kidney Capsule" and the women's is called "Squeezing the Kidney Yin."*

This exercise involves simultaneous movements of arms and legs, as shown in the illustrations. The written instructions here have been divided into the arm and leg aspects. It will take some practice to coordinate smoothly the movement of the four limbs. This is the most difficult and complex exercise described here, so be patient in learning it.

## Opening Posture

Stand straight but not tense, feet shoulder-width apart, arms hanging loosely at the sides. Your gaze is straight ahead (**fig. 1**).

## Arm Aspect of Exercise

Raise the left hand slowly in front of your body with the palm up and the fingers slightly separated, and keep raising the hand along a vertical line in front of the body to chest level. The arms are relaxed and the elbow bends as needed (**fig. 2**).

As you are reaching chest level with the left hand, start raising the right hand in the same type of movement as the left hand, following the same vertical path (**fig. 3**).

The left hand keeps moving up to the level of the head, making an arc to the left side. The eyes follow the left hand. When the hand reaches the level of your head, turn the palm over, fingers curved as if resting on a grapefruit, and move the arm down in a scooping arc (**figs. 4–5**) toward the original position in front of the groin (**figs. 6–7**). Now start bringing the left hand up the front of the body again (**figs. 7–8**).

Meanwhile, the right hand has been following the left in front of the body (**fig. 3**). When the left hand is turning over to begin its downward arc, the right hand is approaching the head level (**fig. 4**). At this time, switch the eyes to follow the right hand as it repeats the movements of the left side, reaching head level

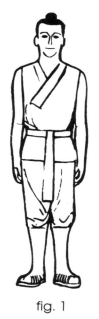

fig. 1

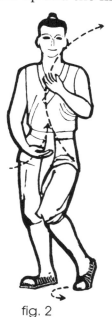

fig. 2

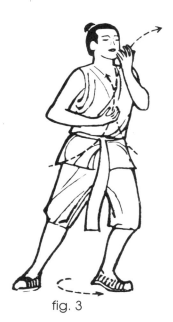

fig. 3

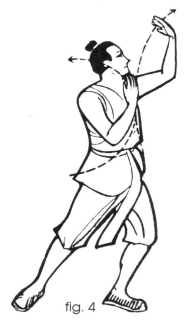

fig. 4

(figs. 5–6), turning over and arcing out to the side (figs. 6–7), and scooping down on the right side (figs. 8–10). While the right hand is making its arc down, the left hand is again being brought up vertically to eye level and you begin to follow the left hand again with your eyes. These hand motions are mirror images of each other.

## Leg Aspect of Exercise

As the left hand moves upward, lift the left foot slightly off the ground and move it in an arc toward the inner side of the right foot, turning the foot so that the left heel turns toward the right foot (figs. 2–3). Keep the thighs pressed as close together as possible. Continue moving the left foot forward and to the left. When it is about two feet away from the right foot, put the left foot on the ground, and shift your weight to the left foot, bending the knee slightly (fig. 4). As you shift to the left foot, turn the body to the left, raising the right foot slightly and bringing it to the left (fig. 5). When the right hand moves to the level of your head, lift the right foot slightly off the ground and move it in an arc toward the inner side of the left foot, turning the foot so that the right heel turns toward the left foot (fig. 6). Continue moving the right foot forward and to the right. When it is about two feet away from the left foot, put the right foot on the ground, and shift your weight to the right foot, bending the knee slightly (figs.

7–8). At this time your left arm is beginning to raise and you are starting the motion of the left foot again (figs. 9–10). The left and right foot movements are mirror images.

## Points of Attention

Hold the thighs as close together as possible during the exercise so that the pubic area feels lightly squeezed. It is important to keep all movements slow, smoothe, and patient.

Once the movements have started, the exercise is done with bent knees. You can decide for yourself the degree of bending which is most comfortable and beneficial. A main point of the exercise is the squeezing of the external genitals between the thighs when the foot turns in its arc. The depth of the squat is less important.

## Caution

Menstruating or pregnant women should not do this exercise.

## Benefits

The gentle, circular movement of the arms stimulates the blood circulation in the arms, increases the elasticity of the muscles and produces smooth comfortable movements in the joints.

Acupuncture points stimulated include: *Waiguan* (Outer Border/Triple Burner—5);

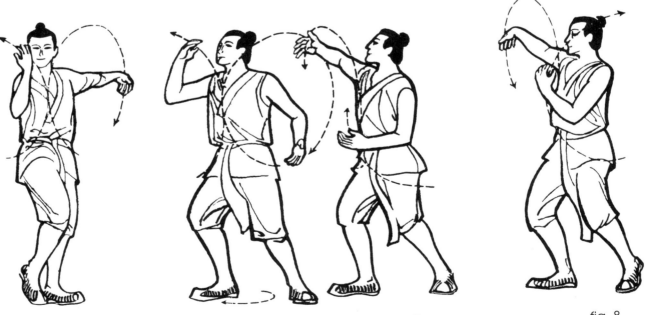

fig. 5          fig. 6          fig. 7          fig. 8

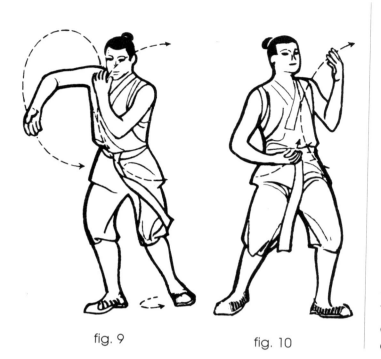

fig. 9          fig. 10

*Neiguan* (Inner Border Gate/Pericardium—6); *Shousanli* (Arm Three Miles/Large Intestine—10); *Quchi* (Crooked Pool/Large Intestine—11); *Jianyu* (Shoulder's Corner/Large Intestine—15); *Huantiao* (Leaping Circumflexus/Gallbladder—30); and *Tianzong* (Heaven's Worship/Small Intestine—11).

Stimulating these points can aid in the recovery from conditions associated with Kidney function in Traditional Chinese Medicine, such as back pain, paralysis of one side of the body, arthritis in the hips, and inflammation of the shoulder joint.

Chinese Medicine sees sagging of the body and organs as due to loss of vitality, which is stored in the Kidney. "Squeezing the Yin" directly increases vitality of the sex organs and can help restore vitality and elasticity to the testicles and the vagina.

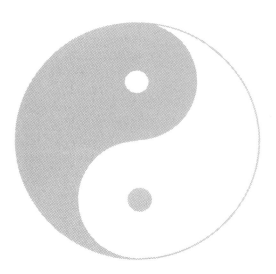

# Exercise 3:  The Eight Diagrams *(Ba Gua)*

*The "Eight Diagrams" refers to the symbol of the yin-yang surrounded by eight trigrams. The trigrams are symbols of various qualities, such as heaven, earth, thunder, mountain, lake. By their arrangement they suggest movement from one quality to another and symbolize internal states of the body and its emotions.*

The arm movements you will learn in this exercise trace the pattern of the well-known yin-yang image (the circle with an S shape dividing the middle into two zones) at the inside of the diagram.

## Opening Posture

Stand relaxed with feet shoulder-width apart, arms hanging loosely at the sides. Look straight forward and try to empty the mind (**fig. 1**).

degrees to the left (**fig. 3**). Bend the left leg more than the right. As the left hand is rising, move the right hand in a downward arc until it is slightly behind the body (**fig. 4**) and below hip level. Then begin moving the right hand up and to the left, drawing a circle to a point above the head (**fig. 5**), turn the palm and bring the hand down to complete the circle. Then, while turning the palm up again, raise the right hand in a curving motion to the left and then right, drawing an S up along the vertical diameter of the circle (**figs. 6–7**).

When the right hand has completed drawing the S, it should be at a point above the head. Turn it downward and draw another circle to the right, around and back up to a point above the head, while taking a step forward with right foot, bending the right knee

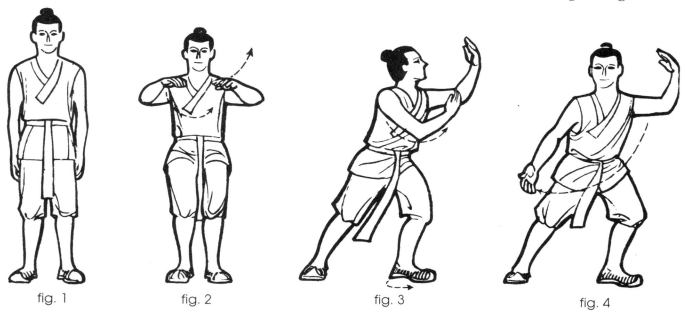

fig. 1     fig. 2     fig. 3     fig. 4

## Movements, Right Side

Raise both hands slowly, palms down as if resting on a beach ball, held apart about the width of the body and bend the knees slightly (**fig. 2**). Keep moving the left hand up until it reaches a point above the head. At the same time, turn the body and the left foot 45

and bending the left knee somewhat less (**figs. 8–9**).

## Left Side

As this right hand circle is being completed and the right hand is reaching a point above the head, you are preparing to draw a

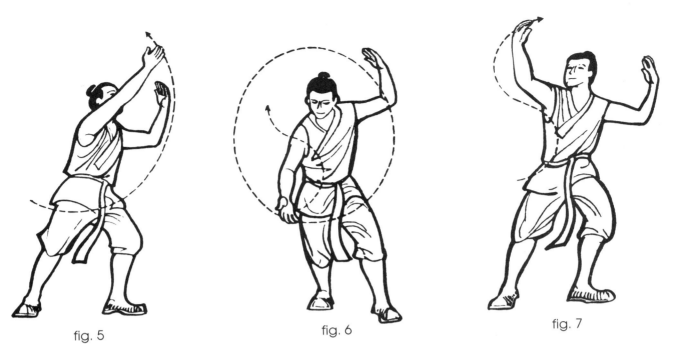

fig. 5          fig. 6          fig. 7

similar pattern with the left hand (**fig. 9**). Turn the body and the right foot 45 degrees to the right and move the left hand in a downward arc until it is slightly behind the body (**fig. 9**) and below hip level. Then begin moving the left hand up and to the left (**fig. 10**), drawing a circle to a point above the head, turning the palm and bringing the hand down to complete the circle (**fig. 11**). Then, while turning the palm up again, raise the left hand in a curving motion to the left and then right, drawing an S up along the vertical diameter of the circle (**fig. 12**).

When the left hand has completed drawing the S, it should be at a point above the head. Turn it downward and draw another circle to the left, around and to a point above the head while taking a step forward with left foot, bending the left knee and bending the right knee somewhat less (**figs. 13–14**). As the left hand is rising, bring the right hand down in an arc and slightly behind the hip to be in a position to begin the right hand exercise again (**fig. 15**).

Keep the two feet close to the ground

fig. 8          fig. 9          fig. 10          fig. 11

and draw the S as accurately as possible. When turning the palm, push out the chest and shoulders. The two hands should be moving smoothly at all times.

Continue repeating the Eight Diagrams pattern, alternating hands in a continuous, smooth manner until you have done the full exercise eight times for each hand.

## Benefits

This exercise is used in China for treating and preventing insomnia, depression, dizziness, and headache. The circling of the arms with the movements of the head stimulate the occiput (base of the skull), increasing alertness and coordination. The movements of the arms increase the mobility of the shoulder joints, shoulder blades, and the neck. The movements of the Eight Diagrams stimulate the following acupoints: *Renying* (Man's Welcome/Stomach—9); *Tiantu* (Heaven's Chimney/Conception Vessel—22); *Quepen* (Empty Basin/Stomach—12); *Fengchi* (Wind Pool/Gallbladder—20); *Fengfu* (Wind's Palace/Governing Vessel—16); *Dazhui* (Big Vertebra/Governing Vessel—14).

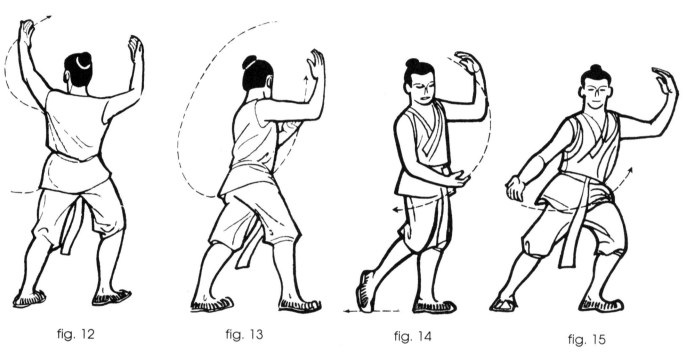

fig. 12          fig. 13          fig. 14          fig. 15

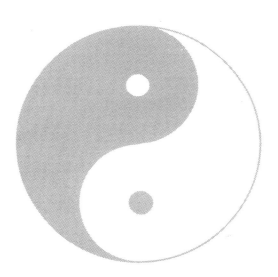

# Exercise 4:   Roc Flying

*The flight of the roc (a mythical bird) is described by tracing a figure eight with the hands.*

## Opening Posture

Stand with feet shoulder-width apart, relaxed, arms at the sides **(fig. 1)**.

## Movements

Push out the chest and pull in the abdomen. Bend the knees slightly and raise the hands, palms toward you, as if holding a beach ball about a foot in diameter **(fig. 2)**. Then, pretend you are rotating the ball a quarter of a turn, so that the right hand is higher, with palm turned down and the left hand lower, palm facing up **(fig. 3)**. While doing this, twist the body and right foot to the right.

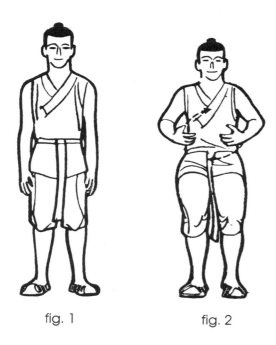

fig. 1          fig. 2

Then, while twisting the body and left foot to the left, bring the left hand up in a circular motion while bringing the right hand down, reversing the position of the hands **(figs. 3–4)**. Now reverse position again by twisting back to the right, bringing the left hand down and the right hand up, palms facing **(figs. 5–6)**.

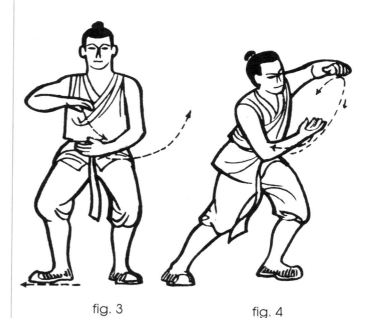

fig. 3          fig. 4

As the right hand begins to return to the starting position in front of the body, it scoops under the left hand and the left hand turns so that the palms remain facing each other.

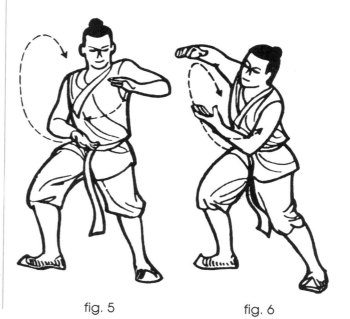

fig. 5          fig. 6

Practice eight complete cycles. The last time, when the right hand returns to the front of the body, let the two hands face each other at chest level and lower the hands slowly and let them return to the starting position, hanging at the sides.

## Points of Attention

Bend the fingers slightly while drawing the circles; stretch the arms outward as far as possible when the hands reach the outer edge of the circle and tauten the back leg. Keep the mind concentrated and the eyes following the moving hands. When turning the body, draw in the lower abdomen naturally. Use a gentle, smoothly flowing motion. The number of times the exercise is done can be adjusted to your physical condition.

As you begin to understand the exercise, you will find that the motion in the waist and arms becomes more fluid, with no starts and stops. The eyes follow the leading hand and the weight shifts over the feet like sand flowing from one leg to the other.

## Benefits

The stretching and twisting of the arms and torso stimulate acupuncture points in the hands: *Shangyang* (Metal's Note Yang/Large Intestine—1); *Shaoshang* (Lesser Metal's Note/Lung—11); *Shaoze* (Young Marsh/Small Intestine—1); and *Hegu* (Adjoining Valleys/ Large Intestine—4), as well as the *Fengchi* (Wind Pool/Gallbladder—20) point in the shoulders. Chinese Traditional Medicine uses stimulation of these points to help strengthen and soften blood vessels in the brain to prevent stroke and headaches.

"Flying Roc" is concentrated at the navel and its twisting motion stimulates the *Mingmen* (Vital Gate/Governing Vessel—4), a point in the spine opposite the navel (between the second and third lumbar vertebrae). Stimulating the navel point will help to keep you centered. The mingmen, which gathers Kidney energy and stores the prenatal qi, will help strengthen Kidney function and can help relieve lower back pain and sciatica.

# Exercise 5: Turtle Retracting Its Head (Multiple Rings)

*In this exercise, the shoulders hunch and the neck stretches and contracts like that of a turtle. The arms describe large circles. The exercise is done at an even, slow speed.*

## Opening Posture

Feet are shoulder-width apart, chest is expanded, abdomen pulled in, and the arms rest naturally at the sides.

## Movements

Slowly raise the arms forward, palms of the hands down, keeping the arms relaxed and the elbows slightly bent. Expand the chest and as the upper part of the body feels lifted, flatten the abdomen. The arms should feel as if they are floating up to shoulder level.

Shift the body weight to the right leg, lean the body forward and turn it slightly to the left. Move the left foot to the left a half step while bending the left knee, and tautening the right leg. At the same time, raise and stretch out the left hand, turning the palm to face the ground. Then bend the wrist but keep the fingers parallel to the ground; while doing this, sweep the right hand downward until the thumb touches the right hip (**figs. 4–5**).

Turn the palm of the left hand outward while raising the elbow outward. Then pull the left arm down and in against the side of the chest (**figs. 6–7**). When making this motion, try to move the shoulder joint in a circular pattern, up, back, and down.

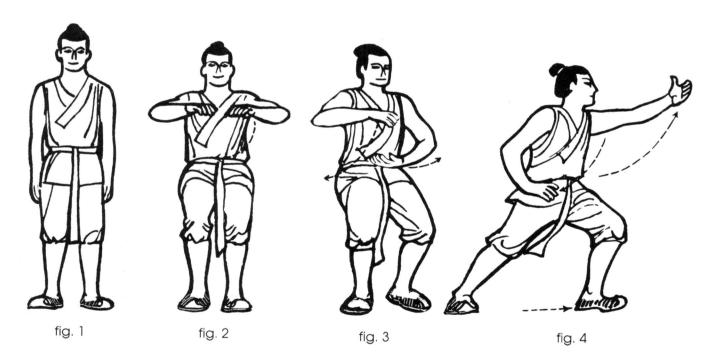

fig. 1       fig. 2       fig. 3       fig. 4

## Left Side Routine

With the left hand, draw a semicircle outward and down to a point near the lower abdomen and turn the hand up as if holding a ball (**fig. 3**).

Now draw a semicircle in front of you with the right hand circling out and up, and bend the right arm close to the side of the chest, bringing it to a position exactly like that of the left, and hold the hand and wrist in the same position (**figs. 6–7**).

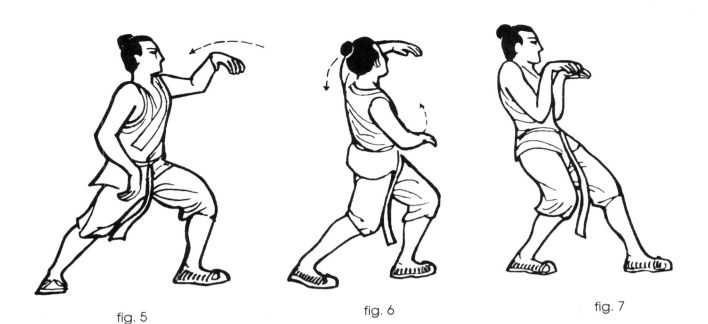

fig. 5　　　　　fig. 6　　　　　fig. 7

Lean the upper part of the body backward, draw in the abdomen, arch the back, and pull in the neck down between the shoulders (**fig. 7**). Rotate the shoulder joints up, back, down, around and forward to a normal position (**fig. 8**).

Draw a large, downward circle, moving both hands down in front of the body almost to the ground and complete the circle scooping the hands forward and up to the front of the chest, pressing the arms against the side of the chest as they were previously (**figs. 9–12**). While making this circle, concentrate on rotating the shoulder joints again: up, back, down, around and forward.

Now begin another large circle in the opposite direction with the hands moving up, forward, down, around almost to the ground and up to the lower abdomen (**figs. 13–14**). As the hands are moving to this position, rotate the shoulders in a circular pattern: up, back, down, around and forward.

Repeat this drawing of circles in both directions, as shown in figures 9–15.

When you have finished these circles and the hands and shoulders have returned in front of the lower abdomen (**fig. 15**), turn the upper body to the right while bringing the left hand up and the right hand down to form the

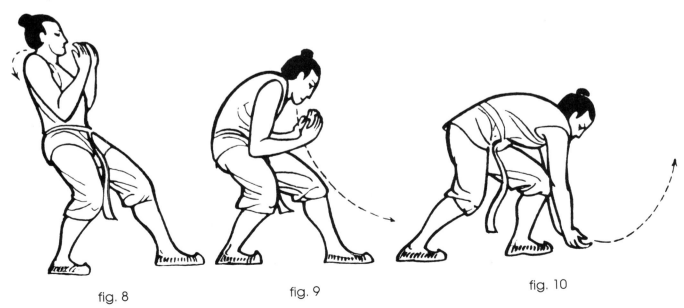

fig. 8　　　　　fig. 9　　　　　fig. 10

33

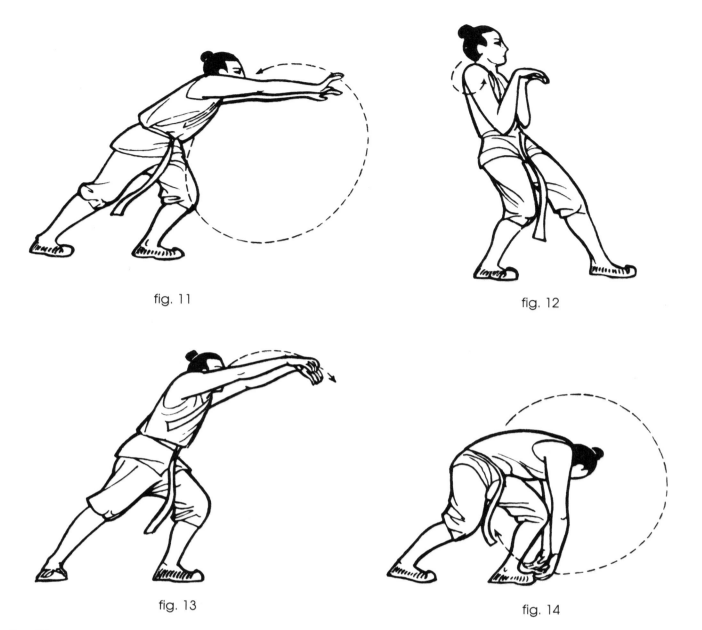

fig. 11

fig. 12

fig. 13

fig. 14

familiar pattern of holding a large beach ball **(figs. 16–17)**. Then shift the weight to the left leg, lift the right leg slightly from the ground and move it half a step forward. Raise and stretch out the right hand while sweeping the left hand downward to the hip. This will place you in the stance shown in figure 18 which will put you in a position to do the right side routine.

## Right Side Routine

The right side routine is a mirror image of the movements of the left side. When you have reached the ending position just described **(fig. 18)**, raise and stretch out the right hand, turning the palm to face the

ground. Bend the wrist but keep the fingers parallel to the ground; while doing this, sweep the left hand downward until the thumb touches the left hip.

Turn the palm of the right hand outward while raising the elbow outward. Then pull the right arm down and in against the side of the chest. When making this motion, try to move the shoulder joint in a circular pattern, up, back, and down.

Now draw a semicircle in front of you with the left hand circling out and up, and bend the left arm close to the side of the chest, bringing it to a position exactly like

34

that of the right, and hold the hand and wrist in the same position.

The next part of the right hand part of the exercise is identical to that for the left hand, as described above and in figures 7–15. Its conclusion is a mirror image of the movements described in figures 15–17.

the neck, chest, waist, and abdomen should form an S shape.

## Benefits

This exercise strengthens the muscles of the arms, legs, waist and abdomen. It is both relaxing and energizing and can alleviate problems of overweight and diabetes.

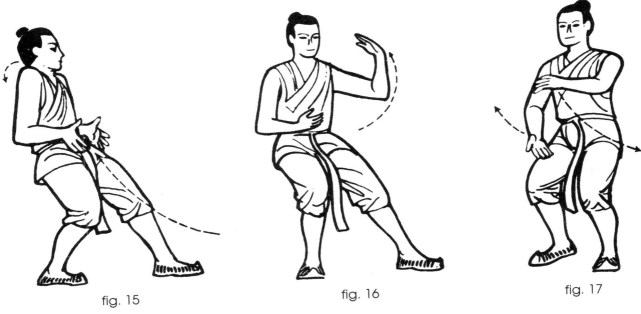

fig. 15          fig. 16          fig. 17

## Returning to Left Position

When you have finished these circles and the hands and shoulders have returned in front of the lower abdomen (**fig. 15**), turn the upper body to the left while bringing the right hand up and the left hand down to form the familiar pattern of holding a large beach ball. Then shift the weight to the right leg, lift the left leg slightly from the ground and move it half a step forward. Raise and stretch out the left hand while sweeping the right hand downward to the hip. This will place you in the stance shown in figure 4, the position to begin the left side routine again.

Do the full exercise, left and right, a total of four times. To conclude the exercise, simply turn the body left and return to the opening posture in a comfortable manner.

## Points of Attention

While drawing circles with the hands, the head and neck should follow the motion of the hands and arms. As always, the movements should be slow, with strong attention to coordination between the shoulder joints, neck and waist. When pulling the arms backward,

The movements of the shoulders and upper back expand and contract the rib cage, increasing respiration and thereby helping prevent diseases of the lung and trachea. The movements of the neck also move the vertebrae of the neck and can relieve pressure on nerves and energize the nervous system. As you make the large circles, you may be able to feel energy moving in your hands and fingertips, indicating that your own energy is flowing smoothly.

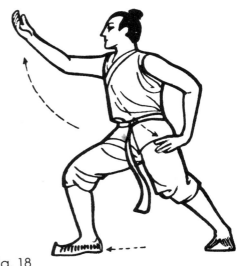

fig. 18

# Exercise 6: The Swimming, Smiling Dragon

*This exercise resembles a dragon swinging its tail as it plays in the water. In one continuous motion the hands trace three circles in front of the body. It begins with a circle around the head and completes the other two circles by making a figure 8 in front of the body. Before beginning, look at the illustrations to get a basic idea of the three-circle pattern you will trace in front of your body with your palms held together.*

Stand with knees straight, and bring the ankles, calves, and thighs as close together as possible. The arms are at the side, the fingers straight and touching each other. Tuck the chin in, smile, and think about being young (**fig. 1**).

With the upper arms pressed against

right hip out to the right while doing this (**fig. 3**). Keep stretching the hands to the left and up with the palms touching. Circle them over the head and down toward the right and in front of the neck to make a full circle (**fig. 4**). (When you make the circle to the left, the right hip swings out, and when circle moves right the left hip swings out). As you begin the down-swing of the circle, your left hand will be on top and the body leaning to the right (**fig. 5**).

Now begin to trace the next two circles as described below and shown in figures 6–13.

Turn the hands over at the chest level, so that the right is on top and both hands are pointing forward (**fig. 6**). Bring the hands out and down in an arc to the left (**fig. 7**). As you bring them back toward the center of the body

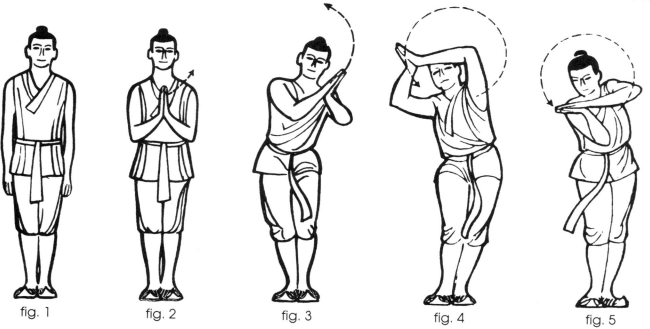

fig. 1      fig. 2      fig. 3      fig. 4      fig. 5

the sides, bring the palms of the hands together in front of the breastbone as if in prayer (**fig. 2**). The hands will stay together in this way throughout the entire exercise.

Begin moving the hands as a unit to the left and up in the first circle (**fig. 2**) while leaning sideways to the left (**fig. 3**). Push the

to complete this second arc, turn them over so that the left is on top and move the hands out in an arc to the right and down (**figs. 8–9**).

As your hands pass through the bottom of this arc (**fig. 10**), turn the hands so that the right is on top, and bring them up and around to the left (**fig. 10**). As you are making this

36

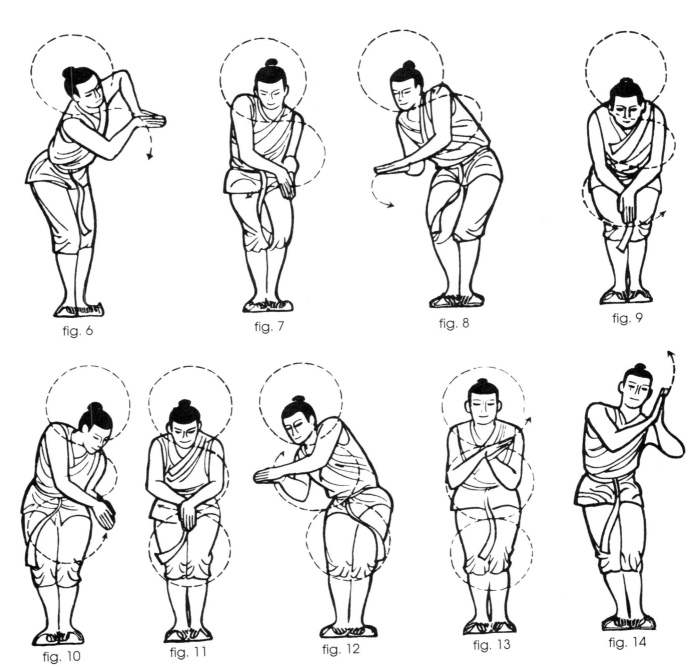

fig. 6　　　　fig. 7　　　　fig. 8　　　　fig. 9

fig. 10　　　fig. 11　　　fig. 12　　　fig. 13　　　fig. 14

second circle, keep gradually raising the body's center of gravity. Continue in an arc up and on the right, bringing the right hand on top of the left and pointing the fingers forward. Continue raising the hands together to the left and up in a circle **(fig. 14)** while leaning to the left. Push the right hip out to the right, continuing to stretch the hands to the left and up, drawing the same circle with which the exercise began **(fig. 3)**.

Repeat this routine four times.

## Finishing Posture

After the fourth repetition has been completed and the hands have come in front of the chest, continue to trace a semicircle up to the left. When the hands are directly above the head, bring them down to the chest and then to the sides in a relaxed way.

## Points of Attention

The circle tracing must be accurate. Be sure to stretch and pull the legs and hips to follow the motion of the hands, moving the hips to maintain the body's center of gravity at different heights. Beginners should increase the width of the hip swing gradually to prevent muscle strain. After a time, as the strength of the waist is enhanced through the exercise, practitioners can trace larger circles with the arms and do wider hip swings.

## Benefits

You will derive the most benefit from this exercise if you can do it slowly and evenly and feel the stretching of the muscles. Practice this exercise as it fits your capacity of movement. As you continue to practice you will find that your knees will bend deeper and your back will be more comfortable as it bends from the hips and reaches into the movements.

The sinuous movements in this exercise limber up the entire trunk of the body because of the twisting at the waist and movement of the torso and shoulders. By toning and strengthening the muscles of the back and increasing the elasticity of vertebrae it helps maintain a straight back even in old age.

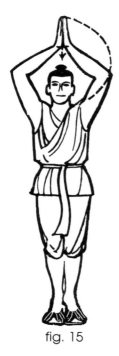
fig. 15

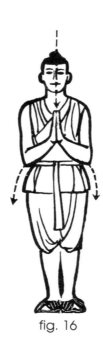
fig. 16

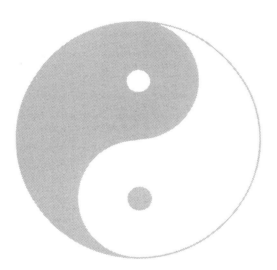

# Exercise 7: Frog Swimming (Small Rings)

*An old Chinese myth describes a golden frog with divine power. This exercise imitates the swimming motions of this frog.*

The opening posture is similar to the Swimming Dragon (Exercise 6). Stand with your ankles, calves and thighs touching, arms at the sides with the fingers touching. Pull in your chin, straightening out the back of the neck, and smile (**fig 1**).

Raise the hands to the chest, so that the palm of each hand is on the chest (**fig. 2**). Elbows are held out to the side and the fingers are held together.

Bend the knees, still keeping them together and shift the weight to the front of the feet. Pull in both the abdomen and neck. Lean forward slightly (**fig. 2**).

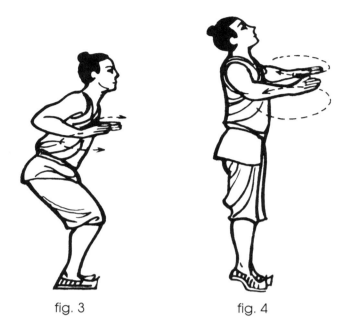

fig. 3           fig. 4

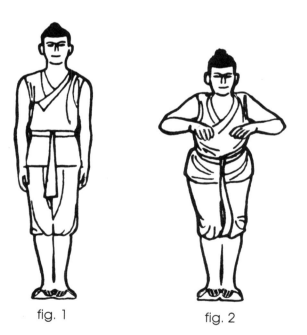

fig. 1           fig. 2

Keeping the hands at chest level, stretch the hands forward and around, making a circle to the outside, and returning to their original position on the chest. As you start to make the circles with your arms, rise up on the balls of the feet and arch the back, push the chin forward and the head back, feeling the neck stretch and letting the buttocks stick out behind. As the arms return around to the chest, come back down on your heels and bend your knees. Do the circles in this direction eight times.

Now, reverse the direction of the circles, moving the hands back and around the outside of the body first and bringing the hands in a circle back to touch the chest (**figs. 5–6**). Rise and lower on your toes, arch the back, bend the neck, and thrust back the buttocks in exactly the same way as for the circles described above. Also do these rings eight times.

## Benefits

Rising up onto the ball of the foot stimulates the *Yongquan* (Gushing Spring/ Kidney—1) point on the sole of the foot.

Moving the neck in and out can alleviate dizziness, stiff neck, tremors in the hands and head, insomnia and amnesia.

Moving the neck in and out also stimulates the thyroid gland and can help treat diseases of the thyroid gland. For those who are recovering from severe illness and are too weak for other exercises, the neck movements will be very beneficial.

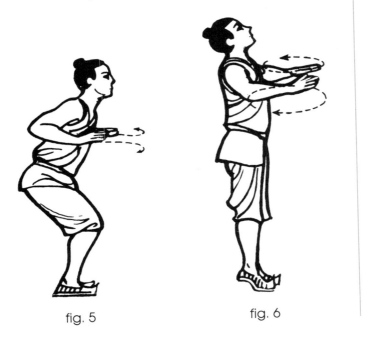

fig. 5                    fig. 6

# Exercise 8: Heaven Circles & Earth Circles

*In Heaven Circles you will trace large circles above the head with the palms turned toward the sky. If you are not strong enough to do Heaven Circles standing, they may be done sitting. If Heaven Circles seem too strenuous or if you have difficulty raising your arms over your head, attempt Earth Circles as an easier alternative.*

## Opening Posture, Heaven Circles

Stand with feet shoulder-width apart, arms hanging comfortably at the sides. Close the fingers lightly **(fig. 1)**.

## Movements

Raise the arms forward, parallel, with palms down **(fig. 2)**. Raise the arms and hands up as far as possible, bringing them behind the head. Describe a large, counterclockwise circle with the hands, bending to the side and back as far as possible without straining **(fig. 3)**.

Do this counterclockwise circle four times. Then reverse directions and make the circles clockwise four times.

As you bend back the hips will come forward. The knees are not really straight, but bend slightly as the trunk moves. Turn the waist first and let the waist movement swing the arms in the circle. The more flex there is in the waist, the more effective the movement. Do not overdo this movement, however.

Let your eyes follow the hand movements and your head follow the arms.

## Benefits

Although this exercise appears simple, it can benefit the lungs, chest cavity, heart and kidneys and can harmonize the energy in the internal organs of the chest, abdomen and lower abdomen (Triple Burner or *Sanjiao* in traditional Chinese medicine).

It is also effective in alleviating dizziness, bad posture, humpback, and sagging breasts in women.

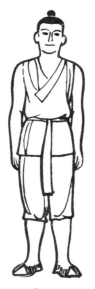

fig. 1

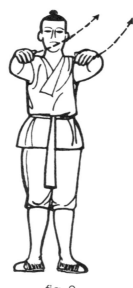

fig. 2

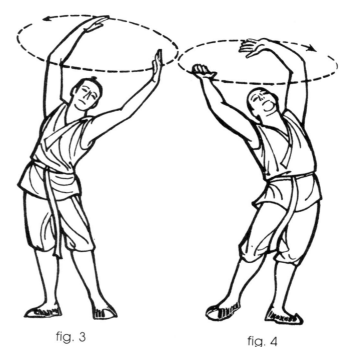

fig. 3

fig. 4

42

## Opening Posture, Earth Circles

Stand with feet shoulder-width apart, elbows held out to the side and hands close to the chest, palms facing the ground (**fig. 1**).

## Movements

Turn the body slightly to the left, shifting the weight to the right foot. Stretch the arms out to the left and at the same time move the left foot about a half step forward. Stretch the hands as far out as possible, reaching out with the upper body, left knee bent, right knee straight, weight shifting to the left foot (**fig. 2**). Then trace a horizontal, counterclockwise circle in front of the body, leaning back on the right foot as you bring the hands around and back toward the chest (**fig. 3**). Trace these circles eight times.

Reverse direction, bringing the right foot forward half a step, moving the hands and outstretched arms in a clockwise circle parallel to the ground (**figs. 4–5**). Trace these circles eight times.

As you make the circles, let the waist turn naturally. Concentrate on describing perfect circles.

## Benefits

Earth Circles is a supplement to Heaven Circles and has the same basic effects.

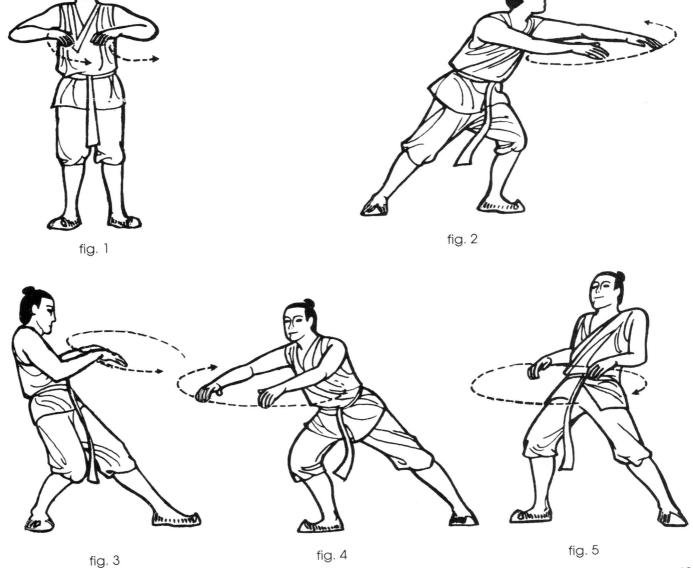

fig. 1

fig. 2

fig. 3

fig. 4

fig. 5

# Exercise 9:  Ren Rings (Cat and Tiger)

*This exercise is a variation of the Heaven Rings. Here you trace five circles in the five directions (north, south, east, west and center). The feet make a pattern resembling the character **ren,** which looks like an upside down V and means "person" in Chinese. Because the movement of the feet is quick and silent, this exercise is also called "cat and tiger."*

## Opening Posture

Standing with the feet shoulder-width apart, slightly bend the knees and let the arms hang loosely at the sides. Face south, looking straight ahead, smile calmly, think of youth **(fig. 1)**.

## Movements

**East** (left):   Raise the hands forward and up, palms facing, elbows bent. Stop  at the point where the elbows are at shoulder level and where the hands are at a level with the *Shenting* (Spirit's Hall/Governing Vessel—24), and turn the palms up, fingers pointing away from the body **(fig. 2)**.

Shift the weight to the right foot and move the left foot about half a step to the left, toes pointing to the left. Moving some of the weight off the right foot, lift the right heel and turn the right heel out about 45 degrees to the left. Turn the body along with the feet, so that now you will be facing left (east) **(fig. 3)**.

Sweep the hands out and downward in an arc and bend forward from the waist as you do this. Bring the palms of the hands together just above *Xiyangguan* (Knee Yang Hinge/ Gallbladder—33) point on the upper part of the left knee **(fig. 4)**. With the hands together and pointing downward, pull them up, close to the front of the body. Pull the body upward and shift the weight to the back (right) foot **(fig. 5)**. When the wrists come to the level of *Shanzhong* point (Central Altar/Conception Vessel—17) on the sternum, rotate the shoulders forward, up, back, and down while turning the hands upward into the praying posture **(fig. 6)**. Separate the hands and push them forward and up in an arc, until the elbows are at shoulder level, palms turned up and fingers pointing outward. While doing this, shift your weight to the left foot **(fig. 7)**. This completes the circle to the east.

**South** (front):  Shift the weight to the right foot and turn the body 90 degrees to the

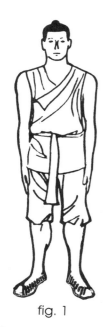
fig. 1

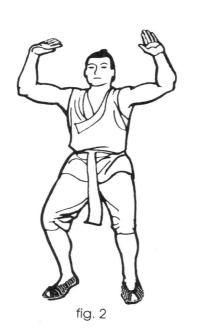
fig. 2

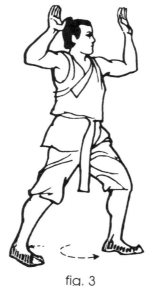
fig. 3

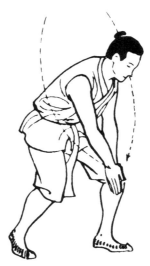
fig. 4

right (**fig. 8**). Pull the left foot in toward the right ankle and then out to the front and left, tracing the upside-down V or *ren* pattern (**fig. 9**). You are now facing south (front).

Repeat the same pattern as you did to the east (**figs. 4–7**). Sweep the hands out and downward in an arc and bend forward from the waist as you do this. Bring the palms of the hands together just above *Xiyangguan* point (Knee Yang Hinge/Gallbladder—33) on the upper part of the left knee (**fig. 10**). With the hands together and pointing downward, pull them up, close to the front of the body. Pull the body upward and shift the weight to

the back (right) foot (**fig. 11**). When the wrists come to the level of *Shanzhong* point (Central Altar/Conception Vessel—17) on the sternum, rotate the shoulders forward, up, back, and down while turning the hands upward into the praying posture (**fig. 12**). Separate the hands and push them forward and up in an arc until the elbows are at shoulder level, palms turned up and fingers pointing outward. While doing this, shift your weight to the left foot (**fig. 13**). This completes the circle to the south.

When you again are standing with your arms to the side of your head, shift the weight to the right leg, pull the left foot in toward the

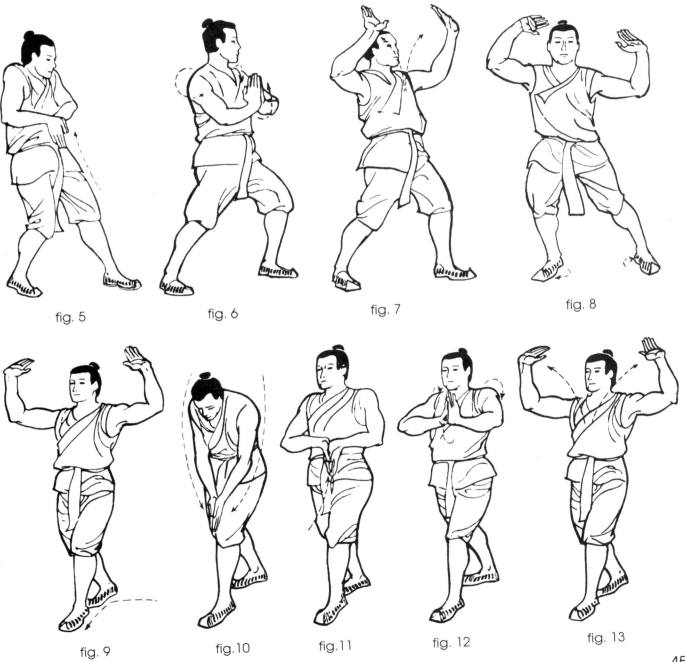

fig. 5        fig. 6        fig. 7        fig. 8

fig. 9        fig.10        fig.11        fig. 12        fig. 13

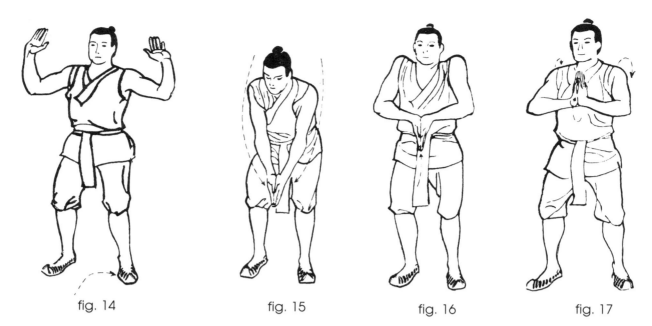

| fig. 14 | fig. 15 | fig. 16 | fig. 17 |

right ankle, and out to the left to trace the inverted V and return to the opening posture **(fig. 14)**.

**Center** (front): The center movement is similar to the first two, with two very important differences. First, the body is squared and feet are shoulder-width apart, as in the posture just described **(fig. 14)**. Secondly, the point where the two hands come together is located equidistant *between* the legs, at the level of the acupoint *Xuehai* (Sea of Blood/ Spleen—10) on the inside of the thighs. (Instead of above the left knee). Otherwise, the

movements are the same as east and south.

Sweep the hands out and downward in an arc and bend forward from the waist as you do this. Bring the palms of the hands together between the legs, at the level of the acupoint *Xuehai* (Sea of Blood/Spleen—10) on the inside of the thighs **(fig. 15)**. With the hands together and pointing downward, pull them up, close to the front of the body. Pull the body upward **(fig. 16)**. When the wrists come to the level of *Shanzhong* point (Central Altar/ Conception Vessel—17) on the sternum, rotate the shoulders forward, up, back, and down

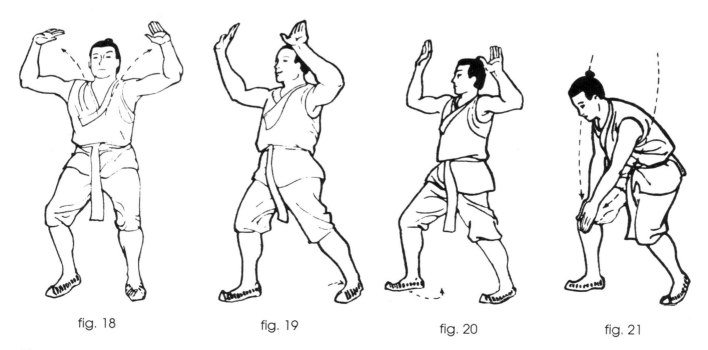

| fig. 18 | fig. 19 | fig. 20 | fig. 21 |

while turning the hands upward into the praying posture **(fig. 17)**. Separate the hands and push them forward and up in an arc until the elbows are at shoulder level, palms turned up and fingers pointing outward **(fig. 18)**. This completes the circle to the center.

**West** (right):   When the center direction has been completed and the hands are again up at the sides of the head **(fig. 18)**, lift the heel of the left foot slightly and turn the heel out 45 degrees to the left **(fig. 19)**. Shift the body weight to the left foot, turning the body 90 degrees to the right. Pull in the right foot toward the left and bring it out again to the right in the inverted V *ren* pattern **(fig. 20)** so that now you will be facing right (west).

The movements to the west are similar to the east and south, except that the *right* foot is put forward and when the hands come together it is at *Xiyangguan* point (Knee Yang Hinge/Gallbladder—33) above the *right* knee.

Sweep the hands out and downward in an arc and bend forward from the waist as you do this. Bring the palms of the hands together just by the *Xiyangguan* point (Knee Yang Hinge/Gallbladder—33) on the upper part of the right knee **(fig. 21)**. With the hands together and pointing downward, pull them up, close to the front of the body. Pull the body upward and shift the weight to the back (left) foot **(fig. 22)**. When the wrists come to the

level of *Shanzhong* point (Central Altar/Conception Vessel—17) on the sternum, rotate the shoulders forward, up, back, and down while turning the hands upward into the praying posture **(fig. 23)**. Separate the hands and push them forward and up in an arc until the elbows are at shoulder level, palms turned up and fingers pointing outward. While doing this, shift your weight to the right foot **(fig. 24)**.

**North** (back):   When you finish the movement to the west, with the arms raised to the side of the head, the weight will be on the right foot. Lift the heel of the left foot slightly and turn the heel out 45 degrees to the left **(fig. 25)**. Shift the body weight to the left foot, turning the body 90 degrees to the right. Pull in the right foot toward the left and bring it out again to the right in the inverted V *ren* pattern **(fig. 26)** so that now you will be facing north.

Sweep the hands out and downward in an arc and bend forward from the waist as you do this. Bring the palms of the hands together just by the *Xiyangguan* point (Knee Yang Hinge/Gallbladder—33) on the upper part of the right knee **(fig. 27)**. With the hands together and pointing downward, pull them up, close to the front of the body. Pull the body upward and shift the weight to the back (left) foot **(fig. 28)**. When the wrists come to the level of *Shanzhong* point (Central Altar/

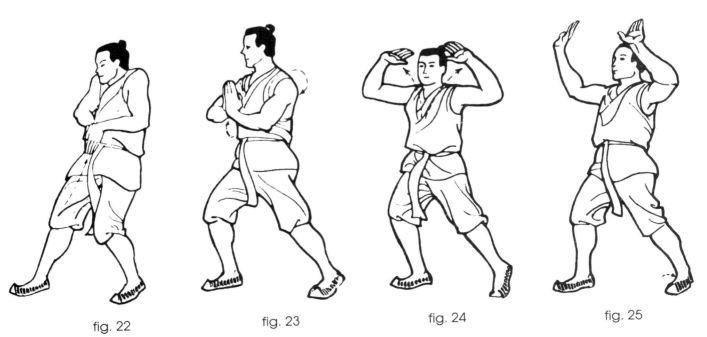

fig. 22          fig. 23          fig. 24          fig. 25

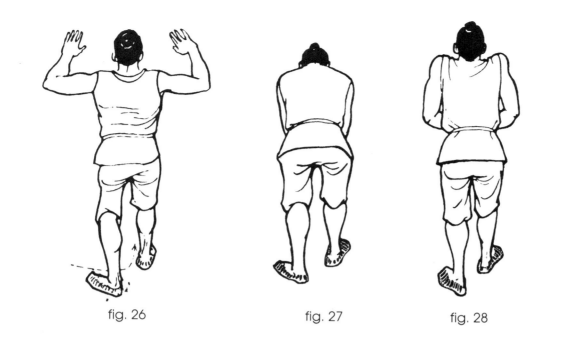

fig. 26       fig. 27       fig. 28       fig. 29

Conception Vessel—17) on the sternum, rotate the shoulders forward, up, back, and down while turning the hands upward into the praying posture **(fig. 29)**. Separate the hands and push them forward and up in an arc until the elbows are at shoulder level, palms turned up and fingers pointing outward. While doing this, shift your weight to the left foot **(fig. 30)**.

This completes the north (back) ring.

To return to the front (south) position, lift the heel of the left foot and turn it 45 degrees to the right, and bring the right foot in to the left ankle and out, making the *ren* pattern **(fig. 30)**, turning the body 90 degrees **(fig. 31)**. Turn the left heel another 45 degrees to the right, shifting the weight to the left foot. Turn the heel of the right foot another 45 degrees to the right, turn the body 90 degrees **(fig. 32)**, and you should be facing front (south).

Lower the hands to the sides as in the opening posture **(fig. 33)**. This exercise can be done several times in a row, but should not exceed twenty minutes.

## Points of Attention

As you become more adept at this exercise, you can begin to add refinements to it. When raising the hands in the beginning posture, you should concentrate intensely, slightly exposing the upper front teeth in a smiling expression. The eyes should have an expression of cat-like concentration.

When you move your feet in the *ren* pattern, feel sure-footed, and move the feet in a steady, quick, continuous, silent motion of a cat.

When turning, bending and stretching during "Ren Rings," pay particular attention to the waist. Feel the waist as the origin of the turning, bending and straightening movements and coordinate the arm and leg and trunk movements with the waist.

## Caution

Pregnant women should not practice this exercise.

## Benefits

The "Ren Rings" exercise was developed according to the theories of yin-yang and the five elements (see Introduction). The goal of this exercise is to amplify the vital energy of the body and extend the life span.

This exercise increases vitality, physical grace, improves the memory, and restores a youthful feeling. Straightening and bending the body, shifting weight and leaning back on the back leg stimulate the nerves that govern the automatic functioning of the body (respiration, heartbeat, etc.) and the sympathetic nerves.

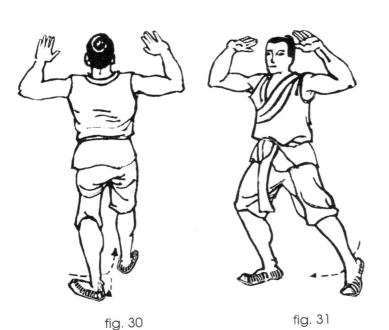
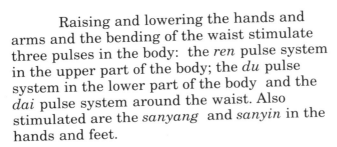
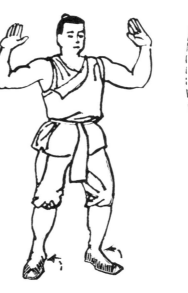

fig. 30　　　　　　fig. 31　　　　　　fig. 32　　　　　fig. 33

Raising and lowering the hands and arms and the bending of the waist stimulate three pulses in the body: the *ren* pulse system in the upper part of the body; the *du* pulse system in the lower part of the body and the *dai* pulse system around the waist. Also stimulated are the *sanyang* and *sanyin* in the hands and feet.

Because this exercise can increase the blood and energy flows, it is used in China to combat the following conditions:

◇ bone spurs of the vertebrae
◇ excessive sweating caused by Kidney weakness
◇ nephritis
◇ numbness in the limbs
◇ lung diseases
◇ bloating in the stomach
◇ pleurisy
◇ hepatitis
◇ intestinal disturbance
◇ breast diseases

The turning movements with the thighs closed squeeze the reproductive organs, helping to regulate and improve the production of sex hormones. In China, this exercise is considered to play an active role in preventing cancer because of the stimulation of the nervous and endocrine systems.

# Exercise 10:  Phoenix Spreads Its Wings

*The movements of this exercise resemble the wing movements of the mythical phoenix. The purpose of the exercise is to relax the mind and body.*

## Opening Posture

Stand with feet shoulder-width apart, arms relaxed at the sides, body relaxed, fingers slightly curved (**fig. 1**).

## Movements

Raise the left hand, palm facing up, to about the level of the navel. At the same time, raise the right hand and bring it, palm facing down, above the left, as if holding a large ball in front of the midline of the body (**fig. 2**).

Raise the left hand while lowering the right, so the backs of the two hands pass each other at chest level (**fig. 3**). Sweep the left hand up and toward the left, with palm upward. At the same time, sweep the right hand down to the right, palm upward. Let your eyes follow the left hand. While making these arm motions, move the left foot half a step to the left, turning the body left and shifting the weight to the left leg (**fig. 4**). As the left hand is approaching its highest extension, turn its palm downward, and as the right hand is reaching its lowest extension, turn its palm upward and away from the body so that the fingers are pointing backward. Turn the head to the right, and look down toward the right hand (**fig. 5**). Feel the stretch from the eyes and neck down to the fingers of the right hand.

Bring the hands back to chest level, so that the backs of the hands pass each other at chest level again (**fig. 6**). Sweep the right hand up and toward the right, with palm upward. At the same time, sweep the left hand down to the left, palm upward. Let your eyes shift to the right hand. While making these arm motions, move the right foot half a step to the right, turning the body right and shifting the weight to the right leg (**fig. 7**). When the right hand reaches its highest extension, turn its palm downward, and when the left hand reaches its lowest extension, turn its palm upward and away from the body so that the fingers are pointing backward. Turn the head to the left, and look down toward the left hand (**fig. 8**). Feel the stretch from the eyes and neck down to the fingers of the right hand.

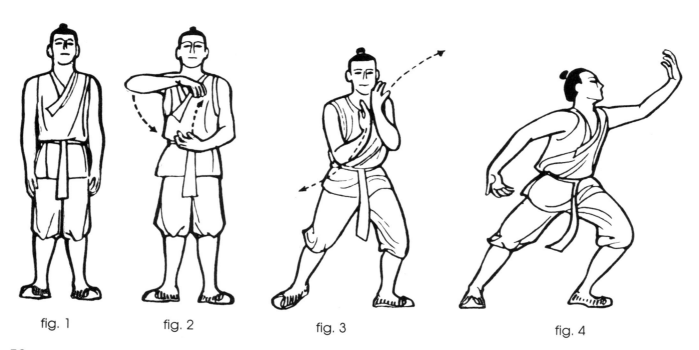

fig. 1          fig. 2          fig. 3          fig. 4

Do four complete cycles.

## Points of Attention

Breathe easily, evenly, and, if possible, into the lower abdomen. The movements should be slow and free, the turning of the body and the changes from left to right hands soft and continuous.

Remember to squeeze the crotch with the thighs when turning the body. Shake the body, arms, and fingers slightly when stretching them. Learning and correctly practicing the "Phoenix Spreads Its Wings" is especially crucial for beginners.

## Benefits

This exercise is the conclusion of the first series of exercises presented here. Its main purpose is to relax the body and serve as the peaceful climax of a series of movements. It harmonizes the energy in the various parts of the body.

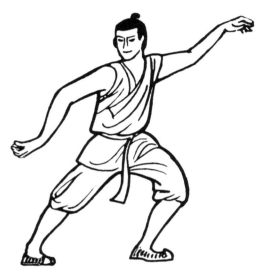

fig. 5

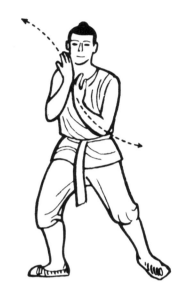

fig. 6

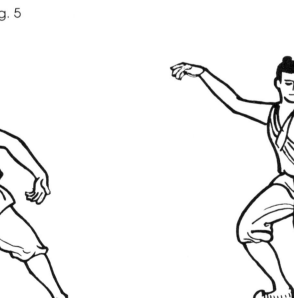

fig. 7

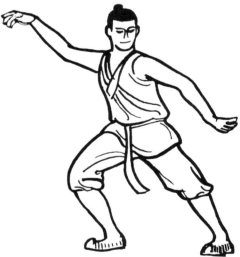

fig. 8

# Exercise 11: Rejuvenating the Face (Moistening the Skin)

*The focus of this exercise is the head, particularly the face. Over time, this exercise will soften the skin, make it smooth and lustrous, erase wrinkles, and prevent growth of skin ulcers and age spots.*

There are fourteen parts to this exercise. The first exercise is to gather earth and heaven energy in the body. The second will direct energy to the hands. The hands are then prepared to transfer energy to

## Movement

Raise the hands, palms facing the ground, arms straight, and bring the hands forward and upward (**fig. 2**). While raising the hands, also begin rising on the toes and inhaling while keeping the abdomen flat. Keeping the arms extended, slowly bring the hands to a position directly over the head. As the hands reach this position, turn the palms up so the fingers point to each other (**fig. 3**).

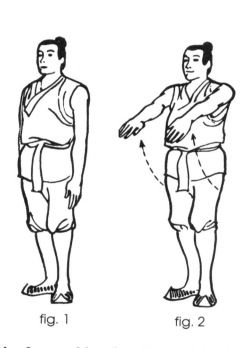 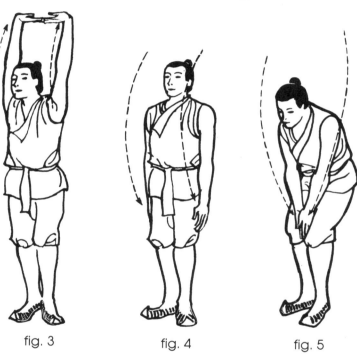

fig. 1  fig. 2  fig. 3  fig. 4  fig. 5

the face and head in the next twelve sections of the series.

## 1) Three Stars High Above

## Opening Posture

Stand quietly with the legs together and toes pointing out slightly. Expand the chest, pull in the abdomen, relax, and let the arms fall naturally at the sides. Breathe slowly and evenly, look straight ahead, smile and maintain a relaxed expression (**fig. 1**).

Turn the hands and lower them, palms down, back down along their original path to the starting position. While doing this, exhale and bring the heels back to the ground (**fig. 4**).

Repeat this routine three times.

## Points of Attention

The Taoists call the inhaled air "living air" and the exhaled air "dead air." This is an effective way to think of the breathing process. In doing the exercise three times, you are re-

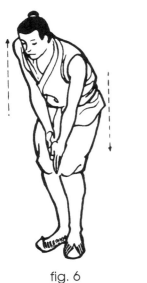
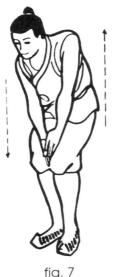

fig. 6               fig. 7

minded of its name, "Three Stars High Above." The first time is called the "Happy Star," the second, "Fortune Star," and the third, "Longevity Star."

## Benefits

According to Taoist theory, *Laogong* point (Palace of Labor/Pericardium—8), at the center of the palm, can attract earth (yin) energy when the palms face the ground. This energy is thought to nourish, invigorate and regulate the blood. Conversely, when the palms turn up, they can absorb heavenly (yang) energy, increasing the vital energy of the body. With diligent practice of the "Three Stars" exercise, blood circulation should improve and yin and yang energy will come into closer balance.

## 2) Sharpening the Eagle's Claw

### Opening Posture

This exercise uses the same opening posture as described in "Three Stars High Above." Stand quietly with the legs together and toes pointing out slightly. Expand the chest and, pull in the abdomen, relax, and let the arms fall naturally at the sides. Breathe slowly and evenly, look straight ahead, smile and maintain a relaxed expression (**fig. 1**).

### Movements

The beginning of this movement is similar to the beginning of "Three Stars Above." Raise the hands, palms facing the ground, arms straight, and bring the hands forward and upward (**fig. 2**). While raising the hands, also begin rising on the toes and inhaling while keeping the abdomen flat. Keeping the arms extended, slowly bring the hands to a position directly over the head. As the hands reach this position, turn the palms up so the fingers point to each other. (**fig. 3**).

Turn the hands and begin to lower them, palms down, back down along their original path. While doing this, exhale and bring the heels back to the ground. As the hands are approaching the hips, bring them toward each other and bring the palms and fingers together as they reach the knees, while bending the knees and waist (**fig. 5**). Insert the hands between the knees (acupoints *Xuehai* and *Ququan*) and squeeze the hands tightly by pressing the knees together (**fig. 5**).

Gripping the hands with the knees, alternately raise and lower each heel, using this movement to cause the palms to rub against each other to generate heat (**figs. 6–7**). Rub the palms together eight times using this motion.

### Points of Attention

This is the key section of the exercise for rejuvenating the face. Do the motion smoothly, continuously, and without overly exaggerated shift of the hands. When rubbing the palms, the fingers should only move along the upper part of each other. The center of the palm (*Laogong* point) should not be moved beyond the outside of the opposite palm.

### Benefits

Rubbing the hands stimulates the acupoints: *Laogong* (Palace of Labor/Pericardium—8); *Yuji* (Fish Border/Lung—10); *Hegu* (Adjoining Valleys/Large Intestine—4), and *Shixuan* (Ten Drainings/Extra—1). The nerves of the spine are stimulated by the shoulder movements.

"Sharpening the Eagle's Claw" can make the finger joints more flexible and elastic and increase blood circulation in the hands. It is also effective in treating headache, toothache, sweaty palms, hysteria, numbness of the wrists and hands, and angina pectoris.

Raising up the heels and lowering them stimulates the foot and leg acupoints: *Zusanli* (Foot Three Miles/Stomach—36); *Sanyinjiao* (Three Yin Junction/Spleen—6); *Dadun* (Great Sincerity/Liver—1); *Pucan* (Servant's Partaking/Urinary Bladder—61); *Jiexi* (Release Stream/Stomach—41); *Chengshan* (Supporting Mountain/Urinary Bladder—57); *Weizhong* (Entrusting Middle/Urinary Bladder—40); *Kunlun* (Kunlun Mountains/Urinary Bladder—60), as well as *Huantiao* (Leaping Circumflexus/Gallbladder—30).

This exercise will also help the hip, knee and ankle joints for those who have difficulty moving, especially in squatting and then coming to standing. It can also combat constipation, pains in the legs, numbness in ankles, pain in heels, foot cramps, and cold feet and legs.

## Caution

Pregnant women should not attempt this exercise.

## 3) Rubbing the Three Phoenixes

After rubbing the hands between the knees, stand up with legs together, continue to rub the palms until they are warm and then cover the eyes with the palms **(fig. 8)**.

Press the palms to the eyes and release the pressure eight times. This motion is called "Rubbing the Phoenix."

Keeping the eyes covered, release the palms so they are cupped loosely over the eyes **(fig. 9)**. Open the eyes and roll them clockwise eight times and counterclockwise eight times. This is called "Turning the Phoenix."

Without moving the hands, move the eyeballs up and down eight times. This is called "Spreading the Phoenix Eyes."

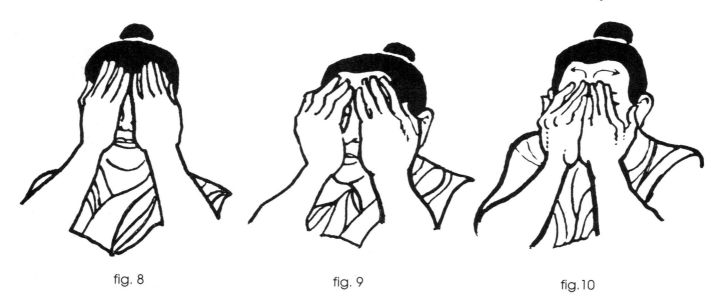

fig. 8          fig. 9          fig. 10

Sharpening the Eagle's Claw stimulates *Huiyin* point on the perineum (Meeting of Yin/Conception Vessel—1) and *Changqiang* at the tip of the coccyx (Lasting Strength/Governing Vessel—1) and pulls at the rectum and gonads. Both stimulate the sex hormones and the movement of the joints can animate the skin cells, increasing their activity to retain freshness of the skin.

## Points of Attention

Keep the hands in the same position while the eyeballs are moving.

## Benefits

Transferring energy from the hands to the eyes and then moving the eyeballs makes this exercise very good for maintaining healthy eyes. It can improve conditions such as: night blindness, cataracts, pain in the eye, near-sightedness, twitching of the eyelid, glaucoma, inflammation of the retina (retinitis), neuropapillitis, and inflammation of the tear glands. It stimulates the eye points *Jingming* (Eye's Clarity/Urinary Bladder—1), *Cuanzhu* (Collection of Bamboo/Urinary Bladder—2), *Chengqi* (Contain Tears/Stomach—1), and *Quihou* (Behind the Ball/Extra—8).

## 4) Replacing Heaven

Using the fingertips of the index, middle and ring fingers, massage along the ridge just above the eyebrows. Start from the the area just above the bridge of the nose and work your way outwards to the temples. Repeat for a total of eight times **(fig. 10)**.

This exercise stimulates the following points: *Tianting* (Heaven's Hearing/Extra—19); *Yangbai* (Yang Brightness/Gallbladder—14); *Shenting* (Spirit's Hall/Governing Vessel—24); and *Taiyang* (Sun/Extra—9).

## 5) Tracing the Phoenix Tail

Place the heel of the hand at the outer corner of each eye. Use the ball of the thumb to rub all the way from the corner of the eye to the temple (*Taiyang* point). Repeat for a total of eight times **(fig. 11)**.

### Benefits

This massage can smooth out crow's feet. It can also relieve conditions such as facial pain, facial paralysis, facial tics, migraine headaches, astigmatism and double vision.

## 6) Tracing Cheeks

Rub the palms to generate some heat, and place the warm palms on the cheekbones. Rub from the cheekbones down to the chin eight times **(fig 12)**.

### Benefits

This massage stimulates blood circulation and cell activity and helps make the skin

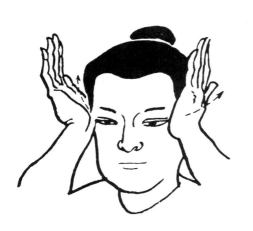
fig.11

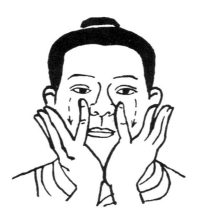
fig.12

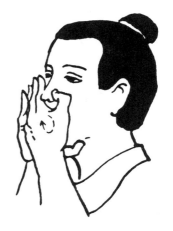
fig.13

### Benefits

This massage can smooth out wrinkles. Stimulating the *Tanting* area can prevent and relieve nasal conditions, tightness or soreness around the eyeball, headache, dizziness, insomnia, high blood pressure, and facial nerve pain (trigeminal neuralgia).

moist, lustrous, delicate and reduces wrinkles and age spots.

## 7) Pressing on the Earthly Store

Stand erect in a natural, relaxed manner. Bend the left elbow to raise the upper arm and place the center of the left palm over the mouth with the tip of the thumb closing the

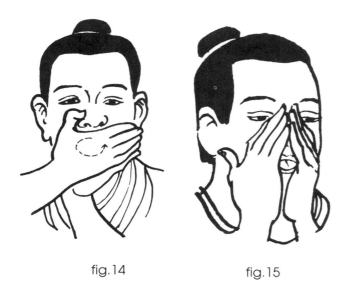

fig.14    fig.15

left nostril **(fig. 13)**. The fingers will lightly cover the right cheek. Bring the right hand up, cupping the chin, and the right elbow placed on the right breast.

Move the hands counterclockwise eight times. As you do this, the left thumb moves rhythmically with the hands, pressing in the dent on the left of the nose eight times. Move the tongue in the same direction as the hands eight times. Coordinate all three movements while breathing in through the right nostril.

Switch the position of the hands and do the same routine, clockwise, pressing the right thumb into the corner of the right nostril,

eight times while rotating the tongue to follow the hands **(fig. 14)**.

## Benefits

This exercise stimulates the points *Dicang* (Earth Granary/Stomach—4); *Renzhong* (Middle of Man/Governing Vessel—26); *Jiache* (Jaw Vehicle/Stomach—6); *Daying* (Great Welcome/Stomach—5); *Renying* (Man's Welcome/Stomach—9); *Xiaguan* (Lower Hinge/Stomach—7), and *Shanglianquan* (Upper Pure Spring/Extra—21).

In China, this exercise is prescribed to prevent and alleviate strokes, facial paralysis, quivering of the lips, unclear speech, excess salivation, mouth ulcers and colds.

## 8) Sticking Out the Tongue

Stand erect in a natural, relaxed manner. Place the hands on either side of the nose and mouth, with the index fingers pressing on both sides of the nose, the thumbs pressing the cheeks, and three fingers over the mouth and nose to leave a little space in front of the mouth **(fig. 15)**.

Open the mouth and stick out the tongue and pull it back. Do this eight times. Then move the tongue freely eight times. Click the teeth together eight times.

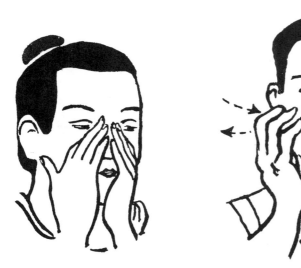

fig.16

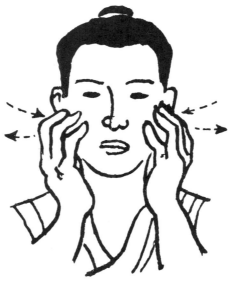

fig.17

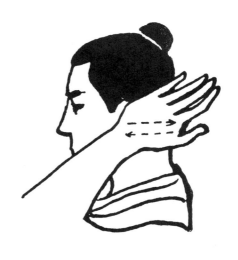

fig.18

## Benefits

This exercise stimulates the nerves in the cheeks and face as well as acupoints *Taiyang* (Sun/Conception Vessel—9; *Xiaguan* (Lower Hinge/Stomach—7), and *Tiantu* (Heaven's Chimney/Conception vessel—22). Because this exercise increases salivation, practice over a period of time can prevent and alleviate dry mouth; it is also used to prevent and alleviate laryngitis, mouth ulcers, tongue cancers and toothache.

## 9) Sucking Jade Liquid

The beginning of this exercise is identical to that of the preceding "Sticking Out the Tongue" **(8)**. Stand erect in a natural, relaxed manner. Place the hands on either side of the nose and mouth, with the index fingers pressing on both sides of the nose, the thumbs pressing the cheeks, and three fingers over the mouth and nose to leave a little space in front of the mouth **(fig. 16)**. Move the lips left and right and up and down eight times. Then close the lips tightly and suck inward. When the mouth is filled with saliva, swallow it. Do this three times.

## Benefits

Do this exercise after doing **(7)** and **(8)** so that you can generate a lot of saliva. Sufficient saliva is important for digestion and Taoists consider it quite significant, calling it "harmony of the vital energy." Tang Dynasty poet Du Fu was referring to saliva when he wrote: "Swallow the liquid of the harmony of vital energy."

## 10) Striking the Dragon's Face

Stand in a relaxed way and rub the hands in front of the chest until they feel warm. Tap the entire face with the finger tips, including your forehead, cheeks, cheek bones, mouth and chin for one minute **(fig. 17)**.

## Benefits

Tapping the face vibrates the nerves of the face and stimulates the subcutaneous tissues to activate the cells and increase blood circulation. This exercise is used in China to prevent and alleviate facial nerve pain, paralysis and quivering. It will also benefit the skin. At the same time, the fingers are also exercised, helping any numbness, soreness, shaking, and coldness of the hands.

## 11) Good Hearing Ears

Stand in a relaxed position and rub the hands till warm. Place the center of the palms over the ears and rub the ears with a back and forth motion eight times, with a little more force going back than forward **(fig. 18)**.

Then, using the middle finger, bend the outside of the ear forward and rest the index finger on the middle finger. Tap down on middle fingers with the index fingers three times, lightly beating the outer ears and ear lobes with a percussive movement **(fig.19)**.

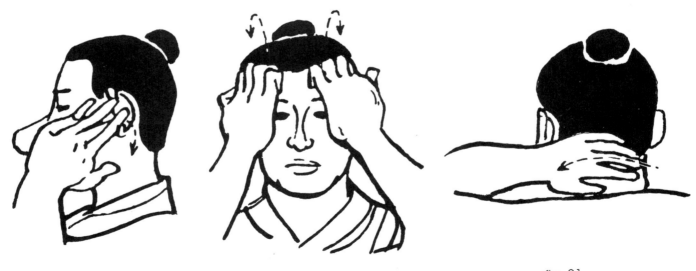

fig.19                    fig. 20                    fig. 21

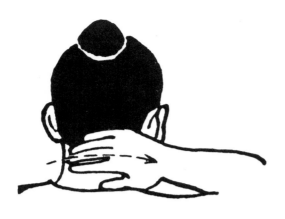

fig. 22

Taoists call this movement "Beating the Heavenly Drum."

## Benefits

Rubbing the ears stimulates the acupoints *Shangguan* (Upper Hinge/Gallbladder—3), *Xiaguan* (Lower Hinge/Stomach—7), on the face and *Tinggong* (Palace of Hearing/Small Intestine—19); *Tinghui* (Reunion of Hearing/Gallbladder—2) and *Ermen* (Ear's Gate/Triple Burner—21) on the ears. This percussion of the ear has been known to help conditions such as tinnitus (noise in the ears), hearing problems and ear inflammation. Tapping the ears can sharpen the sense of hearing, raise the spirits and strengthen the eyesight.

## 12) Rubbing the Dragon's Head

Standing in a relaxed position, use the finger tips and nails as a comb, combing the scalp by pushing all ten fingers back from the forehead to the nape of the neck (**fig. 20**).

## Benefits

Combing the hair with the fingernails stimulates acupoints *Baihui* (Hundred Meetings/Governing Vessel— 20); *Tongtian* (Penetrating Heaven/Urinary Bladder—7), and *Sishencong* (Four Spirits' Intelligence/Extra—1). This may combat dizziness, inflammation of the nose, epilepsy and vomiting.

## 13) Cultivating the Heavenly Pool

Stand erect and put the left hand behind the neck. Rub and squeeze the back of the neck from right to left eight times (**fig. 21**). Switch to the right hand and rub and squeeze from left to right eight times (**fig. 22**).

"Heavenly Pool" is a Taoist term for the back of the neck, including the four points *Fengchi* (Wind Pool/Gallbladder—20), *Fengfu* (Wind's Palace/Governing Vessel—16), *Yamen* (Gate of Muteness/Governing Vessel—15), and *Tianzhu* (Heaven's Pillar/Urinary Bladder—10).

## Benefits

Stimulating these points is thought to prevent and alleviate schizophrenia, pain in the back of the head, involuntary shaking of the head, blurred vision, facial tics and strokes.

## 14) Greater Success

Stand naturally and put the hands in front of the chest. Rub the palms to make

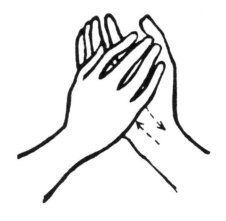

fig. 23

them warm and then rub the center of the palms, backs of the hands, fingers, wrists and arms as if scrubbing yourself in the bath (**figs. 23–25**).

## Benefits

The rubbing of the hands stimulates the various hand points. The exercise is effective for preventing and alleviating excess heat in the hands, sweaty hands, trembling or cramps of the hands, and sore wrists.

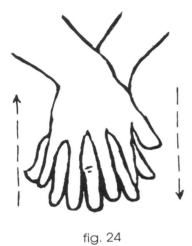

fig. 24

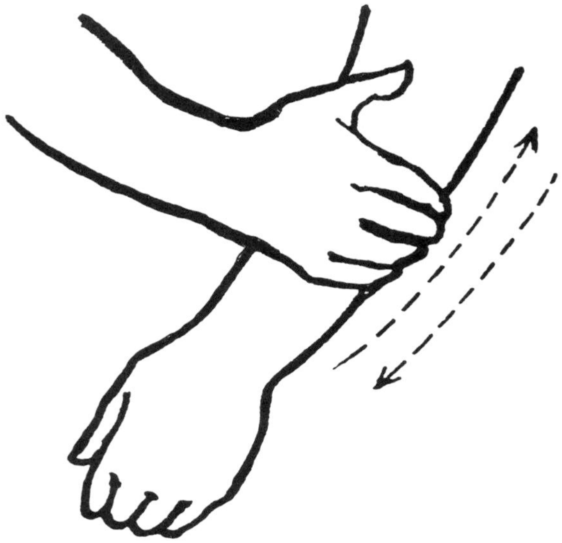

fig. 25

# Exercise 12: Transverse Circles

*In today's society, many more people are spending their workdays in sedentary jobs. After sitting all day without moving much, they frequently suffer tension and pain in the neck and back, sciatica, constipation, and weight gain. Many back problems are due to a combination of poor posture, badly designed chairs, and uncomfortable working positions. Sedentary work is leading to an increase in deformities of the spine, including bone spurs, hunchback, chronic lumbago, and deformities of the vertebrae in the neck. Practicing these sitting exercises can help alleviate these problems. The exercises can be done comfortably in a chair, and can even be carried out while working.*

## Opening Posture

Sit erect and steady, raise the chest, straighten the lower back, keep the two legs and feet closely together, with heels raised slightly. Place the palms of your hands on your knees, straighten your elbows, and feel your chest rise and your spine straighten (**fig. 1**).

## Movements

Focus on your navel area. Move the abdomen and lower back slightly in a small circle around the original point of the navel from left to right (clockwise), up, around and down to where you began the circle. The circle's diameter should be about an inch (**fig. 2**). After making eight of these circles, breathe deeply three times, expanding the abdomen as you inhale and contracting it as you exhale.

Now reverse direction and make eight circles from right to left in a counterclockwise direction (**fig. 3**).

Breathe deeply again three times, expanding and contracting the abdomen as in the first part of this exercise.

## Points of Attention

Relax the entire body to do the movement, making the circles as round as possible, and breathe evenly. It is best to sit on the front edge of the chair, if possible.

## Benefits

Practicing this movement every day can prevent and correct various problems of the vertebrae caused by long-term sitting. It will strengthen your lower back, benefit the kidneys, facilitate the movement of food in the stomach and intestines, promote digestion and excretion, and stimulate the appetite.

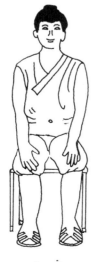

fig. 1

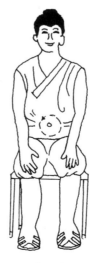

fig. 2

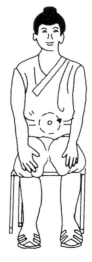

fig. 3

# Exercise 13:  Vertical Circles

*This exercise describes circles turning backward and forward, like a wheel rolling, with the navel at the center. It is similar to Exercise 12, except that instead of describing a circle that moves the abdomen from side to side, these vertical circles move the abdomen up and down.*

## Opening Posture

Sit erect and steady, raise the chest, straighten the lower back, keep the two legs and feet closely together, with heels raised slightly. Place the palms of your hands on your knees, straighten your elbows, and feel your chest rise and your spine straighten (**fig. 1**).

Focus on your navel area. Move the abdomen and lower back slightly in a small circle from the front, down, back, up, and forward, around the point where the navel was when you were sitting still. The circle's diameter should be about an inch (**fig. 2**). After making eight of these circles, breathe deeply three times, expanding the abdomen as you inhale and contracting it as you exhale.

Now reverse direction and make eight circles the opposite way, moving to the front, up, back, down and to the front again (**fig. 3**).

Breathe deeply again three times, expanding and contracting the abdomen as in the first part of this exercise.

## Points of Attention

Concentrate on making the circles as round as possible. The speed of circling depends on individual condition, but it should be slow for beginners. Coordinate the abdomen and lower back movement so that it feels relaxed and natural. Sit near the edge of the chair.

## Benefits

This movement benefits the entire body. It stimulates blood and qi (vital energy), promotes the normal function of the internal-organs, and invigorates the energy that flows in the *Ren,* Conception Vessel, and *Du,* Governing Vessel acupuncture channels running up the spine and down the front of the body.

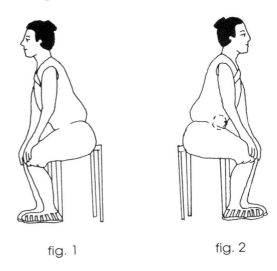

fig. 1          fig. 2

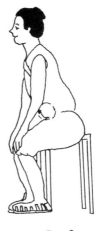

fig. 3

# Exercise 14:   Horizontal Circles

*This exercise describes a circle parallel to the ground, like a plate on a table, that starts by the navel and travels around and into the body and then around and forward to the starting point.*

## Opening Posture

Sit erect and steady, raise the chest, straighten the lower back, keep the two legs and feet closely together, with heels raised slightly. Place the palms of your hands on your knees, straighten your elbows, and feel your chest rise and your spine straighten **(fig. 1)**.

Focus on your navel area. Move the abdomen and lower back slightly in a small counterclockwise circle to the left, around, back, around and forward, around the point where the navel was when you were sitting still. The circle's diameter should be about an inch **(fig. 2)**. After making eight of these circles, breathe deeply three times, expanding the abdomen as you inhale and contracting it as you exhale.

Now reverse direction and make eight circles the other way, moving to the right, back, around, and forward. **(fig. 3)**.

Breathe deeply again three times, expanding and contracting the abdomen as in the first part of this exercise.

## Points of Attention

Regulate the breathing to make it slow and smooth. Do not let the circles exceed an

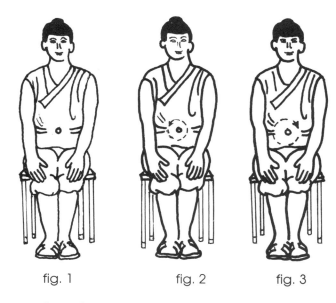

fig. 1            fig. 2            fig. 3

inch in diameter. Keep the movement slow and moderate, so that it can scarcely be observed.

## Benefits

This exercise can help reduce weight and is good for the stomach and kidneys. It's ideal for those who are bedridden and for those who have difficulty walking or standing. Both healthy and weak people can benefit from practicing this movement.

It should be emphasized again that *any* time is a good time to practice the sitting exercises. You can do them as often as you like and under almost any circumstances: while reading, working at a desk, writing, talking or any other times when you are sitting.

# More About the Exercises

Taoist longevity exercises should not be viewed as a cure-all, but as a way of preserving health, slowing down the aging process, and heightening a sense of everyday well-being. The effect of the exercises will obviously be reduced if a person has unhealthful addictions or habits such as smoking, drug abuse, excessive alcohol and caffeine consumption or overeating. A diet deficient in minerals, vitamins and trace elements is also harmful, while excessive fat, salt and sugar have been conclusively proven to be dangerous. Because Taoist exercises use a holistic approach, which takes into account all the elements of health, they are most effective if you are eat and drink in moderation, have well-balanced diet, and avoid stress and fatigue to the extent that you can.

## Fighting Addiction

However, those who do have some bad habits will find that Taoist exercises can be of great benefit in helping to conquer these habits. After all, people resort to smoking, drinking and eating to excess, nicotine and drugs because they suffer from feelings of tension, anxiety, panic, or simply being "out of tune."

Because the exercises restore a sense of well-being and calm, they should definitely be used to help break the cycle of addictive or compulsive behavior. The exercises can help restore the body and mind to a balanced condition that is destroyed by dangerous habits and chemical dependencies. By creating calm, the exercises help ease the uncomfortable feelings which drive people to unhealthful or self-destructive behavior. The pleasant feeling of natural energy in the body brought by controlled breathing, movement and massage can substitute for the "rush" created by chemicals. The restless craving for food and activity can be replaced by a sense of calm and control.

## Sexual Enhancement

All the exercises of the different Taoist schools aim at strengthening sexual organs. Traditional Chinese medicine also uses this theory. Both women and men doing these exercises can develop the power to better control and enjoy sexual activity. Because the exercises open main and collateral energy channels, they can help prevent impotence and increase the intensity of sexual sensations.

Healthy males who have done these exercises for a period of time should find that the heightened body awareness makes it easier to prevent premature ejaculation. Women can strengthen their ability to contract the vaginal muscles, making it easier to reach orgasm. The exercises can help tighten slack vaginal muscles caused by childbirth. Restoring Spring, Vital Energy, Eight Diagrams, Earth Circles, Ren Rings, and Phoenix Spreads Its Wings (Exercises 1, 2, 3, 8, 9 and 10) are especially good for restoring these muscles.

## Help for Chronic Bronchitis, Emphysema and Asthma

Lung diseases are all aggravated by smoking, air pollution and colds. Even healthy lungs lose some elasticity over the years, reducing their ability to expand and contract. Breathing can become uneven and insufficient to fully oxygenate the blood and the cells.

The breathing exercises increase resistance to lung problems by helping maintain the lungs' ability to expand and contract by improving the tone of the muscles used in breathing. Because asthma is often aggravated by stress, all the exercises can help prevent asthma attacks. Those with lung difficulties should devote special attention to Restoring Spring, Vital Energy, Ren Rings and Phoenix Spreads Its Wings (Exercises 1, 2, 9, and 10).

## Fighting Acne and Old Age Marks

With the onset of puberty, hormone secretions increase sharply, stimulating the sebaceous glands. The accumulation of sebum blocks the pores. This, aggravated by bacteria and a bad diet, can cause acne. The exercises can combat acne and other skin conditions such as old age marks by readjusting hormones and improving circulation to the skin. Most effective are the movements of massaging and tapping the face to stimulate blood circulation there (Rejuvenating the Face, Exercise 11). Do *not* expect instant results, however. It is necessary to be quite persistent in improving skin condition.

## Vaginal and Pelvic Infections

Modern medicine can cure vaginal and pelvic infections. If not treated in time, pelvic infection can lead to serious, even life threatening problems. No one with a pelvic infection should avoid medical treatment or attempt to cure it herself. But the use of exercises can hasten recovery and help defend against future attacks.

The swinging, squeezing, and rubbing motions on the sexual organs can increase the secretions of the vaginal wall and strengthen the muscles, building the overall health of the vagina. The same exercises that help enhance sexual experience (see above) will help protect the vagina.

Also, by strengthening the body's immune system through exercises, the chance of infection is reduced. The exercises also stimulate circulation in the pelvic cavity, bringing more disease-fighting antibodies to the infected area. Restoring Spring (Exercise 1) moves the organs of the pelvic cavity up and down. Eight Diagrams, Turtle Retracting Its Head, and The Swimming, Smiling Dragon (Exercises 3, 5, and 6) move the pelvic organs from side to side, creating a kind of gentle internal massage.

## After Childbirth

Many women find their abdominal muscles are quite slack after giving birth. The Swimming, Smiling Dragon movement is effective in tightening and restoring the muscles to their earlier condition. Women who have had a vaginal delivery can begin this exercise in ten days, as long as they do not strain. In the beginning, the movements should be slow and of short duration, with gradual increase. Women who have had a Caesarean delivery should wait until the incision has healed to do the Dragon Swimming movement.

## Correcting Back and Neck Problems

Back and neck problems are epidemic in a sedentary society, and have been aggravated by the widespread use of video display terminals and word processing equipment. Sitting in a static position or constantly hunching and bending over work, causes tension, pain and nervousness that can make life miserable. The cost of medical treatment of these disorders runs into the billions.

The exercises of Turtle Retracting Its Head, Swimming, Smiling Dragon, and Heaven Circles (Exercises 5, 6 and 8) are effective in increasing the elasticity of the back muscles to alleviate tension in the back and neck. Restoring Spring, with its rotation of the shoulders, is especially effective. Cultivating the Heavenly Pool, the neck massage in Rejuvenating the Face (Exercise 11), should also be used to combat neck and back tension. In one way or another, almost *all* of the exercises in this book are effective in relieving spinal problems. As they require no special space or equipment, people with sedentary jobs should do them from time to time during the work day to maintain flexibility, circulation and relaxation of the spine.

## Nervousness and Insomnia

These conditions are perhaps the most common of all. Whole industries have arisen to cope with them. Pharmacists, doctors, psychiatrists, bodywork specialists, chiropractors, and practitioners from almost every branch of the healing arts have been enlisted in this massive war on nerves. The drug industry brings in fabulous revenues on the hundreds of remedies purchased to treat these disorders. Government, university, and private laboratories devote resources to formulating new cures for these ancient maladies. Advertisers and public relations firms make profits marketing each of the new developments to ease this suffering.

The most effective and long-lasting cure for many nervous problems is in the Taoist exercises. In fact, of all the diseases they can alleviate, the exercises are probably most effective against nervous disorders. This is because they induce such deep relaxation if properly carried out. Stress wasn't invented in the modern world. Several thousand years ago, the Taoists discovered that breathing, stretching, movement and massage would reduce the tension that tears at the nerves. Exercising just before sleep or during a sleepless night can produce a deep sleep and a much greater feeling of relaxation the next morning.

## High Blood Pressure, Heart Disease and Stroke

Everyone knows that high blood pressure increases the likelihood of heart attack and stroke, the number one and two causes of death in many nations. Restricting sodium intake will help reduce high blood pressure for many people. Lowering the consumption of saturated fats is now generally thought to reduce fatty deposits in the arteries which clog arteries and bring on heart attacks and strokes.

High blood pressure is very common, especially among middle-aged and older people. The deep breathing and movement in the exercises help relax and expand blood vessels all through the body, lowering blood pressure and improving circulation to the capillaries. The blood supply to the heart itself is also increased. Because of their calming effect, the exercises can be used to combat angina pectoris, shortage of blood to the heart often aggravated by tension and emotional agitation.

## Prevention and Cure of Bone Spurs

Bone spurs can occur as a product of aging, wear on the joints, or injury. They can occur in any part of the body, and are especially painful if they are around the vertebrae. The main

symptom of bone spurs is pain in the affected area.

The exercises can strengthen neck and back muscles and stimulate blood circulation around the joints. With better nourishment, joint tissues grow stronger to support the joints' movements, reducing the incidence of bone spurs. Movements can even help rub or break off the spur, which can then be reabsorbed by the body. One principle here is the same as in Chinese Traditional Medicine, which holds that the Kidney governs the bones, and that bone disease can result from weakened Kidney function. By invigorating the Kidney, the body is better prepared to resist joint problems.

## Arthritis Prevention and Cure

Arthritis is a pathological change in the joints, the causes of which are not yet fully understood, but which involve a complex combination of many factors, including virus, dietary excess or deficiency, injury, aging, exposure to cold, overwork, etc. The main symptoms are degeneration of the surface of joints, accumulation of liquid in the joint cavity, contraction of joint sockets. In the acute stages, the person has fever, feels weak in the limbs, experiences extreme pain in the affected part, along with swelling and intense difficulty in movement.

Medicine and rest are used to treat acute arthritis. Physical exercise can stimulate blood circulation and restore the function of the joints. Arthritis patients should take the initiative in doing exercise even when there is some discomfort. But they should be extremely careful not to overexert. Overexertion will cause negative effects and can aggravate damage already done. Because the longevity exercises are quite gentle, they are especially effective in combating arthritis, as long as there is no straining.

Again, it is best to use the exercises to *prevent* arthritis, by doing them regularly to strenthen joints and improve circulation. The movements break down adhesions in the joints and increase flexibility. The use of the exercises to strengthen Kidney function follows the theory of Chinese Tradition Medicine, which links joint health to the vigor of the Kidney.

# Points Stimulated by the Exercises

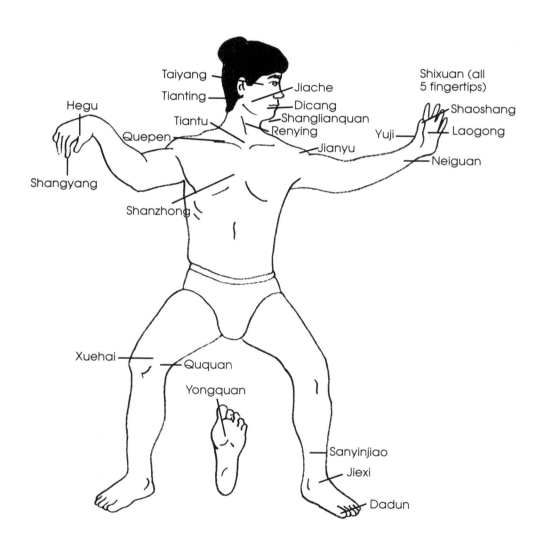

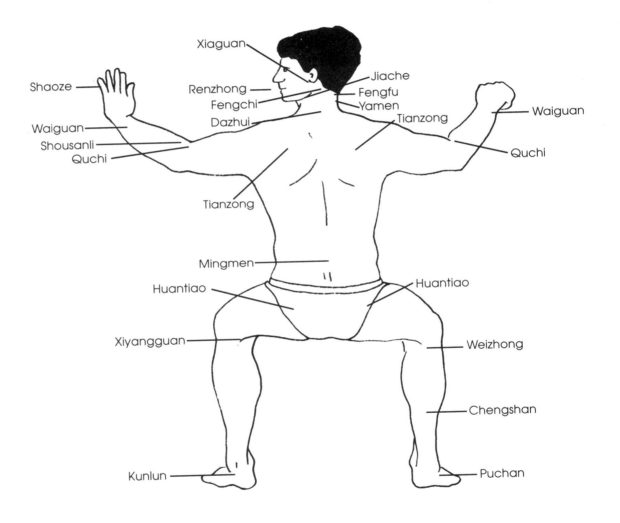

Xiaguan

Shaoze

Renzhong

Fengchi

Dazhui

Waiguan

Shousanli

Quchi

Jiache

Fengfu

Yamen

Tianzong

Waiguan

Quchi

Tianzong

Mingmen

Huantiao

Huantiao

Xiyangguan

Weizhong

Chengshan

Kunlun

Puchan

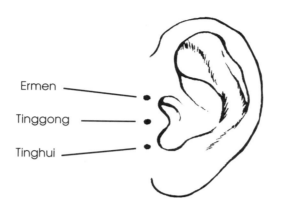

Ermen

Tinggong

Tinghui

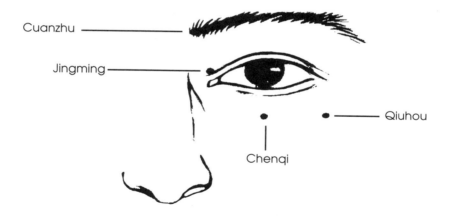

Cuanzhu

Jingming

Qiuhou

Chenqi

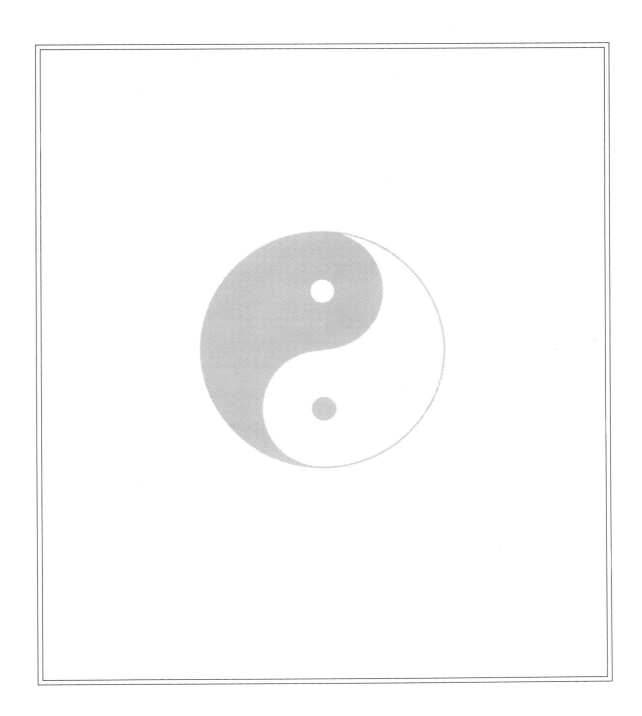

# EASY TAO

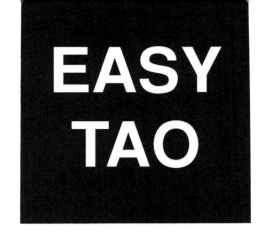

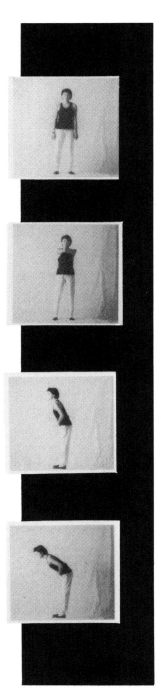

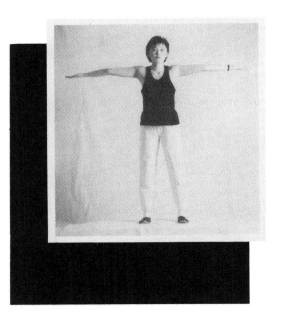

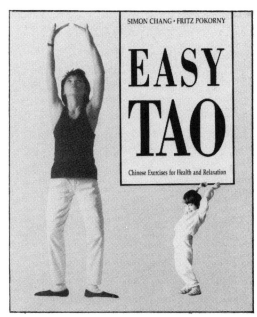

SIMON CHANG • FRITZ POKORNY

## EASY TAO

Chinese Exercises for Health and Relaxation

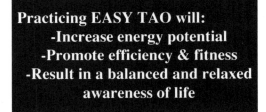

**Practicing EASY TAO will:**
-Increase energy potential
-Promote efficiency & fitness
-Result in a balanced and relaxed awareness of life

For centuries, Qi Gong techniques were held a secret for exclusive use by members of the Chinese imperial family and their friends. Now anyone can experience the benefits of this ancient and powerful method. The twenty basic exercises illustrated in EASY TAO produce a healing energy flow in the body, called Qi, through gentle movements and specific postures. Furthermore, these exercises can be done by people of all ages, with varying regularity and still create successful results! China Books, 1988, 120 pp., 185 b/w photo illustrations, 8 1/2 " x 11". ISBN 0-8351-1833-9................................$12.95

**About the Authors:**
Simon Chang is the director of the Institute of Asian Art in Vienna and former vice-president of the Oriental Culture Study Association of Edinburgh. Fritz Pokorny is an expert on holistic philosophic-physical disciplines and resides in Beijing and Nanjing.

*Send for our mail-order catalog for more listings of health books and China-related titles!*